INNER HARMONY

By Appointment Only series:
Arthritis, Rheumatism and Psoriasis
Asthma and Bronchitis
Cancer and Leukaemia
Heart and Blood Circulatory Problems
Migraine and Epilepsy
The Miracle of Life
Multiple Sclerosis
Neck and Back Problems
Realistic Weight Control
Skin Diseases
Stomach and Bowel Disorders
Stress and Nervous Disorders
Traditional Home and Herbal Remedies
Viruses, Allergies and the Immune System

Nature's Gift series:
Air – The Breath of Life
Body Energy
Food
Water – Healer or Poison?

Well Woman series:
Menopause
Menstrual and Pre-Menstrual Tension
Pregnancy and Childbirth

The Jan de Vries Healthcare series:
How to Live a Healthy Life – A Handbook to Better Health
Questions and Answers on Family Health
The Five Senses

Also by the same author:
Life Without Arthritis – The Maori Way
Who's Next?

INNER HARMONY

Achieving Physical, Mental and Emotional Well-being

JAN DE VRIES

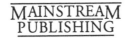

MAINSTREAM
PUBLISHING

EDINBURGH AND LONDON

First published in Great Britain in 1998 by
MAINSTREAM PUBLISHING COMPANY (EDINBURGH) LTD
7 Albany Street
Edinburgh EH1 3UG

Reprinted 1999 (twice), 2000, 2001

ISBN 1 84018 062 5

A catalogue record for this book is available from the British Library

Typeset in Book Antiqua
Printed and bound in Finland by WS Bookwell

CONTENTS

INTRODUCTION

One of the reasons that prompted me to write this book was a gentleman who sat across from me at my clinic in Harley Street. He looked a very ill and very worried man, and he was very hesitant in sharing his problems with me. Finally he plucked up courage and informed me that he considered life was no longer worth living. He confided that he felt suicidal and didn't know how much longer he could last. He was a self-employed businessman and he told me that some time ago one of his best customers had gone bankrupt, owing him more than £60,000, which in turn had caused him to be declared bankrupt. Not only had his business folded, but shortly after that he had lost his only child. A few months later, when arriving home, he found that a number of his household possessions had disappeared. His wife had left him, together with many of their shared possessions, leaving him a note with the message that she would not be back. Somehow, he had still managed to cope, until his only remaining friend, his dog, fell ill and died. At this stage his own health suffered a serious setback and a series of colds developed into bronchitis.

It reminded me of the three bodies of man: physical, mental and emotional, the last of these under more threat than the other two in today's society. When I look at such a suicidal history, I search frantically for ways in which I can help such a desperate person. I started by explaining that any imbalance in the three bodies causes a disharmony in the entire system, which results in physical, mental and emotional pain and anguish. Then it was time to turn to the positive aspects, and I told him that when I worked in China, I had always admired the three temples in Peking: the temples of supremacy, perfection and harmony.

I informed my patient that if these physical, mental and emotional bodies are out of harmony, which was the case with him, the body becomes ill and stressed, and nervous anxiety and fatigue take over. He admitted that this indeed was his experience. I then spoke to him about positive influences, and from recent conversations it is clear that he is gradually becoming a happier person. He has come round to believing that maybe, after picking up the pieces, life may now be better than when he was younger, as he now finds more peace and happiness.

Often in a person's life crises come and go, and whether they are regarded as incidence or coincidence they are part of the forming process of life, preparing us for problems that may arise and, as so often happens, providing us with the knowledge and tools to be of help to others.

In today's society the three bodies of man are under constant attack. Stress has a lot to answer for. Emotional trauma can lead to degenerative diseases, and one must understand the meaning of harmony between left and right, yin and yang, positive and negative.

In writing this book I have drawn on my experiences of forty years with patients, and hopefully the reader may be guided in some of the more difficult situations in life when there is no help at hand. It goes without saying that I have learned a tremendous amount from my patients over all these years, and it is to be hoped that some of my experiences may be of assistance to others when they have to deal with the stressful situations or dilemmas that life has in store for us.

Chapter 1

NERVOUS ANXIETY ~ SELF-CONTROL

Not a single day passes when I do not see several patients who suffer from nervous anxiety. Life today is stressful because of influences on our emotions, and when anxieties get out of control something needs to be done. Unfortunately, many of us are familiar with tension and anxiety, as these feelings are common in our hectic lives. Frequently patients cannot even describe what they are feeling because it is often a gradually increasing pressure, and as long as the anxiety is not too severe, one has the tendency to leave well alone. It may start with being a little impatient. Children or partners are seen as a bit of a nuisance. You may become irritable and find it difficult to concentrate. Stress often expresses itself in insomnia: either not being able to fall asleep, or being unable to remain asleep during the night. Small issues and not being able to deal

with the demands of your job can cause an unrealisti-
cally high degree of anxiety. Physically, the effects of
stress can result in constipation, diarrhoea, sexual problems, aggressive tendencies, insecurity, rapid heartbeat,
headaches or dizziness.

Whatever the cause or the symptoms of the anxiety, it
can be dealt with in many ways. Some people benefit
from gentle relaxation exercises, relaxing body and
mind, while others find relief in hard physical exercise.
As each individual is different, instinct often tells you
what is most suitable for you, because the body's own
way of coping with such a situation is usually the best.
However, there is no value whatsoever in telling someone that he or she will just have to learn to live with it.
A person suffering from anxiety needs help, because the
condition is more likely to deteriorate than improve. It is
advisable to act at an early stage and develop a measure
of self-control over your state of mind. Sometimes an
anxious mind can cause pain and discomfort, and this
should be recognised as a warning signal. Please do not
sit back and let it overcome you, but take determined
action before it is too late.

Patients are sometimes curious to know if I have ever
suffered from nervous anxiety, and I am the first to
admit that, of course, I have had my disappointments
and moments when life did not come up to expectations.
In many instances, my experiences with patients have
provided me with valuable information on how to cope
with my own anxiety.

If we want to master anxiety we must first know
something of its nature and ask ourselves what nervous
anxiety really is. The question is simple enough, but not

so the answer. Even psychiatrists and psychologists cannot quite agree on this. We know that the brain receives a great number of nervous impulses, some of which are conscious and others that are subconscious. The impulses arise from different areas: from the external environment, from the body itself and from the mind. The information concerning the external environment comes to the brain via our five senses. We are well aware of the sensations and a great deal of subconscious information comes to the brain from all parts of the body. This is an extremely complex process, and it can cause a lot of problems and conflicts. The impulses from the environment, the body and the mind are integrated, and negative impulses often become too much to cope with. The body's response to anxiety can be many and varied. When our heart rate increases, blood is diverted and blood pressure rises, and this is a sure sign that the body is preparing itself for action or flight.

The body has many self-regulating mechanisms, for instance those that control body temperature, fluid balance and the chemical concentrations in the blood. When the sympathetic nervous system becomes very active, a self-regulating mechanism calls the para-sympathetic system into action to balance the effect of the over-active sympathetic system. The brain has a major task to perform. When more messages arrive than the brain can handle, we approach a state of anxiety. The level at which this happens varies according to the individual. Our mental ability may become stressed by the situation and in its mobilised state the mind becomes unusually alert, often too alert, and then develops a pathological over-alertness which becomes so active that even an unexpected noise could affect our situation.

This over-alertness shows itself in many ways. When a person becomes distressed, the anxiety sometimes becomes so dramatic that self-control is easily lost. At this stage a person may act out of character, as his or her common sense is affected. Unfortunately, in some cases the anxious state has progressed this far because all warnings have been ignored. We are often reminded of nervous tension we have experienced before, and most of us are familiar with the obvious signs. Anxiety will manifest itself in a multitude of ways, however, and some of these are of such a nature that we are often misled by the symptoms.

In one of my clinics I saw a young woman in her mid-thirties who told me that her doctor had diagnosed her as suffering from nervous anxiety. She informed me of her symptoms in a slightly agitated manner, but she was nevertheless very descriptive. She explained that when awakening in the morning she often had butterflies in her stomach. She did not feel like getting up and the thought of yet another day was enough to depress her. She felt incompetent at work and worried that she would be unable to cope. Anxious about the future, she asked me for advice. She had told me about her symptoms, but I chatted with her in order to find out more about the underlying problems. We discussed some relaxation exercises and a low-stress diet avoiding products with a high protein and high fat content. Furthermore, I recommended that she take Dr Vogel's Centaurium, twice a day, fifteen drops before meals, together with two Neuroforce tablets after meals twice a day.

Somewhat to my surprise, she told me that she had read about Centaurium but had always understood that it was designed to combat loss of appetite and stomach disorders. She was indeed well informed, but I reassured her that she too would benefit from a homoeopathic solution of Centaurium. Centaurium also has an effect on the vegetative nervous system, which lies below the navel. Especially when incorrect breathing is involved, the vegetative nervous system can become very tense, and problems such as those my patient had described can be experienced: feeling uncomfortable, feeling tired, butterflies in the stomach. Often the metabolic system is also involved and help is necessary in order to regain the balance. Centaurium contains the extract of cornflower and is a very useful remedy to settle problems of the vegetative nervous system. At her third visit to the clinic my patient told me with a laugh that the butterflies had left her stomach.

Once she felt more relaxed, she admitted that initially she had been very apprehensive and that it had taken a lot of effort to pluck up the courage to make an appointment to see me. This is not unusual in cases of nervous anxiety, as one of the symptoms of the condition is that people can become very apprehensive about new experiences and making decisions. There is a fear of the unknown, and patients are often afraid of sharing or discussing their problems with others.

There is actually a considerable difference between nervous anxiety and nervous tension. True apprehension is an indication of nervous tension, where relaxation is necessary. Very often nervous tension expresses itself in the manner of irritability, insomnia, fatigue, depression, lack of concentration, difficulty in communicating, phobias and phobic tension, obsession, restlessness, stuttering and other similar symptoms. Symptoms of nervous anxiety, on the other hand, are palpitations, slow and fast heartbeat, nervous dyspepsia, constipation, possible impotence, headaches, and so on. The common causes of anxiety present themselves in several ways. A disharmony between the three bodies often displays itself in marital and sexual problems, aggression and insecurity.

Nervous anxiety is an immense problem, and many people have difficulty controlling this without help from outside, i.e. taking medication, adopting a low-stress diet and exercising self-control. So many people come to me having been to the end of the road and gone through all the channels, and are then put off by the simplicity of my treatment. Once they start, however, they see how much better they feel and how little it takes to be successful in overcoming nervous anxieties.

POSITIVE SELF-CONTROL

Every molecule, every atom of this universe, animate or inanimate, is in constant vibration. Each mineral and each living cell in man, animal or insect vibrates on its own frequency and wavelength. There are also vibrations of sound, colour, smell – and heat and light. In addition, the earth and all its living things are continuously being bombarded by stellar vibrations and cosmic rays of a frequency too high for us to comprehend. Furthermore, the earth is surrounded and criss-crossed by magnetic bands, man-made radio currents. All is vibratory in nature. These are facts and governed by law.

Vibrations of sound can cause pleasure or pain, according to their effect on our emotions. The rhythmic tune will start our feet tapping involuntarily, while a plaintive melody will often cause tears or a lump in the throat. A dog will cry out in pain at the blast of a whistle and will howl painfully at the strains of a violin. There is also power in the human voice, power to influence or to offend. The ancient peoples knew of the power of the spoken word, as is clear from the old proverb 'A soft answer turneth away wrath'.

Most powerful of all, yet least understood, are the cosmic vibrations. That they exercise a profound influence on our lives cannot be doubted. The energies are there, constant and powerful. It is up to man to harness and use these forces to help himself and his fellow men. Man is a complete entity in himself: body, mind and soul.

Throughout the universe, fatigue is the only thing that invariably leads to distortion and destruction. The human body is no exception to this. In such cases the joints become strained, and skeletal relationships are changed. Muscles operating around such joints are stretched. The alkalinity of the body is lost because of fatigue toxins becoming acid in reaction and the cellular structure loses its potential. By analysing the distortion and applying certain rules, the body can be realigned, the distortion corrected and the destructive change stopped. Only then will the alkalinity be restored and health rebuilt.

One must remember that the force of gravity affects everything, and the study of the human body from this approach is the main theme of this teaching. The four main essentials underlying the preservation of life are food, temperature, rest and elimination. All these factors depend on gravity in its last analysis.

Few men, even those whose business is the study of physics, have understood gravity so well as to grasp the idea that every other law is the outgrowth or manifestation of the fundamental law of gravity. The first attraction that forms a nucleus, and the attraction of a nucleus for its electrons, is through the various chemical reactions made possible by the atoms thus formed. Every force and every energy is directly resolvable for its reason to this law. This force that we call gravity – every source of power, electricity, mineral and vegetable – is only a manifestation, or another phase, of gravity.

The fact is that energy exists in matter in some form or another. It is this ever-present energy that causes both chemical and physical change. Heat alone is sufficient to produce physical change in matter, by altering the form of the energy contained therein, and it is manifested in a change of molecular structure.

In fact matter, almost without exception, can be changed by the addition or subtraction of heat alone. The three phases of change are:

1. Gaseous
2. Liquid
3. Solid

These are the most easily demonstrable states in which matter exists, but each of these three states is again found in either a colloidal or a crystalloidal state. A true colloid with all its very definite properties may be converted by external agents.

The tissues of the body are largely colloidal, and the human body and its diseases are our present concern. Because of this it is necessary to understand the action of colloids and the forces that change them into crystalloids. This change manifests itself as disease. All pain and every abnormal condition of the body is the result of this change.

All living matter has what we call life force. Colloids are extremely sensitive to the action of external agents, due to the softness of their gelatinous colloid particles. Life of the cell depends on the creation and maintenance of an electrical potential, and the various functions of life are due to variations of that potential. Living cells are self-charging condensers built on the fundamental plan of the atom. The solution is the colloid. Electricity is the thread which binds together form and function.

In the human being we find the most positive cells in the brain and its appendages. These cells form the positive pole of the body. The liver is the negative pole of the body because it collects waste products.

The human machine is composed of three parts. First there is the skeleton of bones held together by the ligaments in such a manner as to provide joints. Muscles are applied to introduce motion into these joints and nerves are applied to control the action of the muscles and the blood vessels, thus providing a source of nutrition and waste removal. The second part is the great mind of man, that gift of God that makes us potentially different from our fellow creatures. The third part is the extremely delicate processing and manufacturing plants which are contained within the body and usually designated as the viscera. This processing plant is designed to take in a variety of raw materials and to convert them into products usable by the various components of the manufacturing division. These three parts, while often separated into items for the manipulator, psychiatrist and physician respectively, are actually welded into a single functional unit by the autonomic nervous system.

The autonomic nervous system, with its chemical counterpart the endocrine system, constitutes the great two-way street by which the three major components of the body are tied into a fundamental and functional unit. Anything, large or small, which happens in one part will be reflected in one or both of the other parts. The general attitude has been a tendency to limit thinking to two parts of this human machine, the mind and the viscera, while ignoring the mechanical and electrical phase. The three should always be considered as a whole, however, as is taught in the sensory motor technique, the triune polarity of existence.

The nervous system performs all the functions of the body. If the motor system is disturbed, excessive or deficient action ensues. Disturbance of the sensory system may result in pain. The sympathetic nervous system is the superintendent of all bodily functions, and we must seek always to establish the circulation of the blood and other fluids. We provide the mould for the creative law, and unless the mould is increased, the substance cannot increase. Man is fundamentally made perfect; disease has no location, no expression.

Every time we think, we are thinking into a receptive,

plastic substance which receives the impression of our thoughts. When we stop to realise how subtle thoughts are, how we unconsciously think negatively, how easy it is to become down and out, we see that each man or woman is perpetuating his or her own condition. This is why people go from bad to worse, and from success to great success.

It must be understood that all diseases have a common origin and that this origin is a toxic condition resulting from food fermentation – from life to death. This original cause has a major influence upon the condition of a patient. Often symptoms are frequently examined and treated as the cause. A fast will often cure a disorder, for the simple reason that fasting gives cells of the body a chance to get rid of these toxins. Within every man and woman is a force which directs and controls the entire course of life. It can heal every affliction and ailment to which mankind is exposed.

Energy must flow. Any sore spots are blocks in this energy current at either the positive, negative or neutral poles. One must first locate where this energy block exists and, on discovery, release it. When these triune body currents are re-established, the pain will leave at once and normal activity can take place.

In dealing with the body's magnetic fields, whether it be for diagnosis or for treatment, the north versus south position is very important for the positive axis of the body. The east versus west position is equally important for the circular axis or the magnetic waves around the long axis. In magnetic healing, it is believed to be best for a patient to be placed with his head facing north in order to get this long axis sweep. Success depends on this long axis and local polarisation of the patient's own fields, by releasing the sympathetic spasm which is usually located in the sympathetic nervous system.

There are billions of cells in every square inch of tissue in the human body. These cells have an inbuilt intelligence. These cells breathe and excrete waste matter and can even live independently of the human body – and indefinitely. When the Creator gave man his perfect body, he also gave him a complete set of controls to keep this body in perfect order and harmony. Viruses and germs do not cause our aches and pains, or deficiencies and infections. These can never really harm a body that is in a healthy state. Man is a balanced creation of physical, mental and spiritual attributes.

It was said by a great philosopher, Hermes, the Thrice Great, 'Everything flows out and in; everything has its tides; all things rise and fall; rhythm compensates.' The very same principle manifests itself in these positive, negative and neutral poles, even when we go through the necessary process of breathing. Correct breathing is a major aspect of positive self-control, and to this end breathing exercises can be extremely useful.

Man seems to be the only creature who is not aware of what he is doing or where he is going. Ants and bees, for example, have an advance knowledge of the part they are destined to play throughout their lives. We lack the knowledge of the physiology of the nervous cells, and how the mind is influenced by the state of the organs. It often looks as if man has his priorities wrong; remember that mystical laws became known long before those of physiology.

There is a reason for the slow progress of knowledge of

ourselves. The life of small groups has been substituted by the herd. Solitude is looked upon as a punishment, and sometimes as a luxury. Modern civilisation seems incapable of producing people endowed with imagination, intelligence and courage, and discoveries are developed without any consideration of their consequences. Man is actually becoming a stranger in his own world.

There is, however, a possible remedy for this evil, and it rests in a more profound knowledge of ourselves. The science of man has become the most necessary of all sciences. The proposition that man is composed of matter and consciousness is really meaningless. Every body is animated by an invisible power, and this makes the body possess the qualities of a magnet.

Ultimately, it is of no use for us to increase the comfort, the luxury, the beauty and the complications of our civilisation. All this will prove of no value if our weaknesses prevent us from guiding this knowledge to our best advantage. The science of man will, and must be, the task of the future. Soul and body are creations of our methods of observation. The human body is far too complex for us to apprehend it in its entirety. The quality of any individual partly depends on that of his surface, as the brain is continually being moulded by the messages it receives from the outer world. Let us always bear in mind the saying 'Man Know Thyself'.

Some time ago a young couple brought their ten-week-old baby to me. Due to the death of a close relative during her pregnancy, the young mother had lived through a very stressful period. The birth of the baby was difficult, resulting in a forceps delivery. The mother was obviously very upset when the newborn baby had its first epileptic fit. The fits became worse, and when drugs did not seem to help, the parents brought the baby to me.

As I have done with my own children and grand-children, I always look first, immediately a baby is born, to see what the breathing is like. This breath that God gives a person to enable him or her to be a living soul is perfect harmony in a baby. Right under the navel, which is the last tie to the mother to be broken when the cord is cut, lies the centre of harmonious breathing. There is no better sound than the wonderful harmonious breathing of a newborn baby, which will change as the child grows up. Unfortunately, when a baby becomes nervous, its breathing becomes more shallow. It no longer follows what we call the Hara breathing method, from right underneath the navel, that is of such tremendous influence on the vegetative nervous system.

This little baby still had good breathing, however, and that was the reason why I was optimistic. I had to apply a small cranial osteopathic adjustment right on the top of its skull, where the forceps had been applied to the cranium. It took no more than a few seconds, but that was all that was needed. There has not been another fit since.

I also advised the mother that in order to help the baby to balance its energy she should put its left hand on its stomach and cover this with its right hand. This would help the baby to relax, and I recommended that she teach this to her child as it grows up. This simple act of placing the left hand below the navel and placing the right hand over it whilst breathing gently relaxes a person and is of great help for positive self-control. When I heard how positively the child had reacted to the cranial adjustment, I was so grateful to the Creator of all life for giving us the means to regain harmony. I was also grateful to my teacher, Denis Brookes, who is a great cranial osteopath, who taught his students: Find it, fix it and leave it.

Positive self-control can be greatly helped by placing the hands on the stomach, in the way described above, and breathing slowly in through the nose, into the stomach, and then exhaling through the nose. This method of relaxation, known as the Hara breathing method, as well as many others, is described in my book *Stress and Nervous Disorders*.

A little while ago I saw a gentleman who had first had an appointment some three months previously. At that time he was very stressed and he confided in me about his fears, worries and anxieties. The only advice I could give him was that he had to learn to relax, learn to value life and learn to live it to the full. I told him that harmony in the body was of the greatest importance, and therefore the first requirement was that he had to change his diet. He was on a very high-protein diet, which is always bad – but never more so than for someone who suffers from stress. I asked him to cut out high-protein foods such as meat and eggs, and to introduce more rice and complex carbohydrates. I also asked him to try and give up alcohol. I taught him the Hara breathing exercise and gave him some simple advice to overcome his insomnia. I prescribed two Neuroforce tablets to be taken twice a day after meals and twenty drops of *Avena sativa* to be taken before meals, again twice a day. Finally, I suggested he carry Emergency Essence in his pocket, as in stressful circumstances flower essences can be of great help. When I saw him again recently he was anxious – anxious to tell me how very much better he felt. We should all learn about the importance of inner harmony and how it can be achieved physically, mentally and emotionally.

Chapter 2

DEPRESSION ~ HUMOUR

There are many forms of depression, and it is for psychiatrists to define the kind of depression they are treating in order to determine the best approach. Depression can be caused by anxiety, alcohol abuse, neurosis or psychosis, resulting in reactive, masked or endogenous depression or dementia. Depression can strike unexpectedly, where previously there has been no problem, and can easily ruin a person's life. Patients often ask me in wonderment why they should be suffering from depression. They claim never to have had any problems before and then, because of an accident, misfortune or disappointment, they are at risk of being caught in this downward spiral.

The mind, that second part of the human machine, plays a great role. Full of frustration, fear and other mental stages, it finally ends in crystallised matter at the negative pole which is the pelvic basin. The energy distribution between mind and coccyx is carried out by the glandular areas. These whirl from the right like a spinning-wheel and increase in their circumference, energising the right and the left of the body. If there is harmony between left and right, there is health and rhythm of life. Mental upsets, dietetic errors and many other factors thrust upon us by modern civilisation prevent this in varying degrees. The life force gets blocked in various ways – and when it gets blocked entirely, death is the result.

The basic premise in all healing methods is to understand fully the whole human being. Many thousands of words have been written on this topic, some confusing, some enlightening, some not making any sense. Man has been endowed with the faculties of a mind, a body, a soul and a heart (or spirit). Being enclosed, these faculties expand to give man the different states of mental, physical, spiritual and emotional expressions. The live human being must expand further to utilise these expressions by thinking, by looking around and observing, by acting on the information gathered and by feeling a sense of completeness. As each square expands, it gives man the ability of fulfilment, alters his general appearance, enables him to communicate and then helps him to develop an attitude to his whole existence and environment. Man can work through fulfilment or hold an introspection by moving inwards to understand himself.

Each body cell is composed of atoms, is bi-polar, has a nucleus of solar electricity and is dominated by magnetic force. The polar properties of attraction and repulsion of the cells are very marked. They unite and separate in exactly the same way as do two electrified bodies, and that is what they are. Two other functions are expressed by the cell, i.e. volition and sensation. Volition is the power of selection and rejection. Sensation is the power of response of sensitiveness to impressions.

These four fundamental functions of the cell result from the action of solar force on the poles of the cells, producing all phenomena summed up in the word 'life', with each organ and gland performing its allotted work. Here, under the very nose of the scientist, we have Carrel's 'Unknowable Reality', Osler's expression of 'a series of chemical changes', Spencer's 'continuous adjustment of internal relations to external relations', and Bichat's 'sum of the functions (of the body) by which death is resisted'. There is that mysterious life principle which scientists are unable to find or define, because they do not know what they are searching for. Creative processes present these four fundamental functions which are inherent in the atom and appear in the body cells in the form called life.

Psychologists ask whether there is mind power, termed subconscious or subjective, that is not limited by time. Many things appear to indicate that there is. The ancient masters believed that there is, and set out to prove it in their work.

The principle of polarity in the human body is the action of the finer energies in nature which work like the atomic energy on wireless waves. The radiant waves of this innate energy of life and warmth sweep over every living cell as an attraction and repulsion current which is the prime mover in embryonic cellular life long before there is an organised telephone system of nerve tracts for specific function and action. This primary motive energy of life is a triune principle in operation as male (positive) and female (negative), or a neutral pole (child or product), as well as the unknown origin of both poles in the beginning. So, the first is the last in the process of creation in all forms.

It is only through the discovery of atomic action that we can be convinced of the actual presence of this function in every particle of matter, including the human body. This warmth of life, like the atomic heat, is then stepped down and transmuted into chemical and mechanical action guided by sparks or nerve energy to control its local and specific function. These finer forces in nature were seen as realities by the ancient masters. They are the key to the principles of health and its application in the body through manipulative polarisation, the lost art of healing.

The neutral position of the embryo in the mother's womb helps to build the body by these finer energies in nature's secret domain prior to chemistry and mechanics. The energy pattern and the geometric designs created here carry on through life and build the nervous system, the circulation, the glands and the muscular and body structure to express its own latent pattern and desire.

The body of man is a microcosm in a macrocosm and is thus subject to all the physical, chemical and electrical laws that govern the universe. Recent moon probes have shown that the earth has not only an atmosphere but also an ionosphere surrounding it. Different layers, which are fine electromagnetic energy fields, surround the earth. What happens in the ionosphere finally takes place in our atmosphere. There is concern about what is happening to our protective ionosphere. Hydrogen and atom bombs have ruptured our protective ionosphere, allowing the ultra violet and cosmic rays to penetrate, and this, in time, will injure our vegetation.

If you wonder what this has to do with the electro-magnetic field of our bodies, remember that the body is an extension of the earth. We have three finer magnetic fields:

1. The electrical magnetic field
2. The mental electrical magnetic field
3. The emotional electrical energy field

Actually, the entire universe constitutes a mass of electro-magnetic light waves in gravitational movement. In other words, the universe, including the human form, is continually in a state of pulsating electromagnetic light waves as solid and liquid gases, but in reality these waves are continually manifesting themselves as motion or vibration.

Disease means dis-ease, or lack of ease or harmony, or the lack of well-being. Emotion means a moving-out of energy. These energy fields have to be normalised or balanced before the disease or symptom can be corrected. Disease is really the result of disorganised electrical forces, and we must learn to organise these forces in order to be in good health.

When the three electrical magnetic fields mentioned are out of harmony, depression can set in. It should be remembered that the body needs ninety-one nutrients, and one missing nutrient can result in a disturbance in this electromagnetic field. This is the reason why patients with anorexia nervosa or bulimia are subject to depression. The lack of only one mineral such as zinc can turn a healthy person into an emotional wreck. It is of the utmost importance that harmony is restored as quickly as possible.

A youngish girl from the very north of Scotland came to see me. At nineteen years of age she was a sorry sight: depressed, and bordering on the verge of anorexia. When I tried to find out about her background I learned that she was the only daughter of a very strictly religious middle-aged couple. In their love for her they had sheltered and over-protected her. Not being allowed to mix with others from her age group, and therefore lacking mental stimulation, she had slowly become depressed. In her depression she paid no attention to her diet, and this in turn had caused havoc with her health, due to a major imbalance of vitamins, minerals and trace elements. I was pleased that this girl had come to see me, because she confided in a gentle manner and explained about her parents' convictions without accusing them. We discussed how she should slowly adjust her lifestyle, without upsetting her parents, by leading a more normal life and achieving mental stimulation. This was the foundation for her return to health, and it was underwritten by prescribing zinc, a vitamin complex and Concentration Essence. She occasionally writes to tell me that she is happy. She has balanced her background and her future, has developed a great love for classical music and has turned into a voracious reader. She now lives in peace with her religion.

Then I am reminded of a young married woman who was deeply depressed when she came to see me, so much so that she was actually unable to speak. To give her time to collect herself I took a blood sample. I soon discovered a large number of deficiencies, and it was obvious to me that a poor diet was having a detrimental influence. When we discussed her condition I soon learned that after the loss of a member of her family she had lost interest in everything and as a result had paid no attention to her diet, which had been the last thing on her mind. Once on the spiral of deterioration and depression, she sank lower and lower. In such cases Zincum valerianicum has always been a tremendous help (fifteen drops twice a day). Fortunately this lady took my advice, and within a few weeks there had been a remarkable improvement. At her last visit she brought me flowers and was delighted to inform me how happy she was.

This brings me to the story of St John's wort. When I left the Netherlands some thirty years ago to make my home in Scotland, I brought with me ten litres of Dr Vogel's Hypericum Complex. This is a fresh plant extract made in Switzerland. As it was impossible to bring a wide variety of remedies, I felt that this would be one of the best for me to bring for my first patients in Scotland. Hypericum Complex, a very diverse remedy, is beneficial for circulatory problems, and over the years my faith in it has been confirmed time and time again. It is a remedy that lives up to its signature and characteristics. It gives great encouragement. When looking at the design of veins on a leaf of St John's wort under the microscope, it is reminiscent of the intricate nervous system. The leaf is full of little holes, hence the name *Hypericum perforatum*, or St John's wort, and it has been a blessing to countless patients.

Recently, at a lecture, I was handed a newspaper article written by a psychiatrist in which I read that *Hypericum perforatum* was as effective as Prozac in the treatment of depression. I smiled, because I remembered how some time ago I wrote about St John's wort in a series of articles that featured in several national newspapers. Suddenly there was a flurry of research and several companies brought out products containing hypericum. For more than forty years I have prescribed *Hypericum perforatum*, and in my mind it is an outstanding remedy. Not only is the plant attractive to look at, I feel that it almost shouts out that it loves us (hence its less formal name of St John's wort). Like many natural remedies, hypericum has been overlooked for many years, being viewed as unfashionable. Fortunately the clock has now been turned back and it is again widely used. I should, however, add that in my opinion the fresh extract made into such a wonderful formula by Dr Vogel is still one of the best.

Some time ago I was delighted to receive a postcard from a female patient who was touring India. When she first came to see me she told me about her life. She had lost loved ones and possessions, and was severely depressed. In this state she had lost interest in life and as a result had developed an alcohol dependency. Eventually she had also become addicted to drugs. When I first saw her I decided on acupuncture treatment to try and regain harmony in the electromagnetic fields, and I also applied osteopathic treatment. I prescribed Emergency Essence, and gradually she began to climb out of her depression. It did not happen overnight, but eventually she managed to overcome her addiction to drugs and alcohol. I was so delighted to receive that postcard, because to me it was once again confirmation that with positive steps depression can be overcome.

Laughter is a great medicine. I remember once, after a spell of extremely intensive studying, arriving at my grandmother's, quite depressed and miserable. She instructed me that every day I should try to sing a song and look for something to make me laugh. She insisted that laughter is the very best medicine of all. It may be worth remembering that it takes only fourteen muscles to smile, but that seventy-two muscles are required for a frown. According to my wise grandmother, one stands to lose everything if one loses humour in life. I agree, because over the years I have learned that humour is one of the best ways of combating depression.

At a lecture I referred to my book *The Five Senses* and was asked if there might be a sixth sense. I spoke about the five tangible senses while referring to a possible sixth sense, intangible but nevertheless real. This is a sense that mainly functions by smell, enabling us to smell situations and possibly alerting us to the unexpected. When I finished the lecture, a lady drew my attention and stated that there was also a seventh sense which I had not mentioned. When I asked her to explain, she pointedly stated: 'A sense of humour.' She was right, of course, because although this is a sense which we easily forget about, a sense of humour is of the utmost importance. Too often we take ourselves too seriously, neglecting the lighter and brighter side of life. In my practice we are used to dealing with illness and disease, but thankfully we are not devoid of humour, and that is what keeps us going. I know only too well that when one is depressed the last thing one thinks of is humour, and yet a good joke can make all the difference. In this respect I have found that the flower essence of the Californian wild rose, *Rosa californica*, has often been of great help. The flower's signature is that life is to be enjoyed, and this rose carries the message of the beauty of life added to humour.

Although I do not often accept lunchtime engagements, on one occasion I made an exception. By popular request I had been invited to give a talk at a Rotary Club luncheon and immediately afterwards I returned to the clinic to start a very busy afternoon surgery. My first patient that afternoon was a dear old lady who had been a patient of ours for a long time. She was a farmer's wife who suffered greatly from osteo-arthritis, particularly in her knees. When she felt really in need, she would phone to make an appointment for acupuncture treatment, and that way we managed to keep her going. She was a gentle and pleasant person, never very demanding, which especially endeared her to the staff. Always very punctual for her appointment, she also showed great appreciation for the relief of her pain after the visits.

This afternoon, as always, she was wearing her little bonnet, which, by the way, she never took off for her acupuncture treatment. I remarked that she was looking a bit pale that day and she told me that she had been very busy and had also been off her food. We chatted away while I positioned the acupuncture needles, and I also checked her blood pressure and her heartbeat. Nothing out of the ordinary was found. I then looked in on another patient, leaving my principal physiotherapist in charge. Shortly afterwards I was called back, as she was not happy with the old lady's condition.

I immediately realised that our patient was about to faint, and although we took preventive action, she went out like a light. When I took her pulse again it was only slight and my physiotherapist could not locate anything stronger. We were baffled and becoming increasingly concerned. We had just reached the decision that an ambulance should be called when she opened her eyes.

Now, imagine this dear little face, with the bonnet still planted on her head, albeit slightly askew, as were her spectacles. There was not much of her, but she looked even more frail lying there, with the colour drained from her face. When she opened her eyes, she asked in her kind and gentle voice, 'Is that it for today? It seems to have gone so quickly.' She actually sounded disappointed and clearly had no idea how much anxiety she had caused, being totally unaware that she had passed out during the treatment. Not noticing the beads of perspiration on our faces caused by our frantic efforts to revive her, she remarked with a friendly smile that it had been a very good treatment today and that she felt very relaxed.

We helped her up and explained to her what had happened. She then apologised for all the trouble she had inadvertently caused and we took her to an ante-room where she could have a quiet cup of tea. Having heard what had happened, she was ready to accept our advice that she must take things a little easier and take better care of herself. Some of the work would just have to be left until another time, and she had to slow down a bit. Don't we all, when growing older, have to accept the fact that we are not spring chickens any more and therefore do not have the physical stamina of an eighteen-year-old?

As I said earlier, humour is one of the many ways to overcome depression. Indeed, it is a very important one, together with the remedies that I have mentioned. Remember the ninety-one nutrients required to keep a healthy mind in a healthy body, and this may prevent depression from developing into a chronic condition.

I witnessed a good example of humour when working in Northern Ireland. While working in my surgery, I heard yet another bomb explosion. As always I was shocked, as it reminded me of my youth, growing up in the Netherlands during the Second World War. The bomb squad came, cleared the area, and life went on. The positive attitude of the people of Northern Ireland and the silent hope that one day this would all pass ex-pressed itself when, a little later, one of the officers who was involved in the clearing up of the debris asked my receptionist for an urgent appointment. During the clearing-up operation he had hurt his neck by a careless movement. He asked me to treat him and when we were ready he smilingly gave me an example of the positive attitude of the Northern Ireland civilians. Apparently, while he was removing the debris an old lady passing by asked him for particulars. She mumbled in response, thanking God that it was not thunder or lightning, and went on her way. This positive approach I have often come across in the years I have worked in Ireland, and the attitude of these people has often been a great encourage-ment. It is heartwarming to witness such a positive attitude in a situation of distress.

Laughter is definitely the best medicine. This is now widely recognised, and I have learned that courses are available for practitioners in order to help people to regain their sense of humour. It gives great satisfaction to get a laugh from a depressed person. The best possible outcome is if we can persuade people to laugh about themselves, because with a sense of humour we can conquer the world.

Chapter 3

JEALOUSY ~ ACCEPTANCE

enjoy the sight of my seven grandchildren playing together. On one occasion they were having a wonderful time until one of them came to sit on my lap and spontaneously gave me a cuddle. After a few minutes, one of the others approached slowly and hinted that she was also there, and of course I gave her a cuddle too, under the watchful eye of the first. Fortunately there was no rivalry. I thought, though, how often in such situations we see little flashes of jealousy, between children and adults alike.

Often I have had patients who were secretive and even untruthful in their answers until I discovered that they were jealous. The reasons could be material or resulting from a relationship, and this jealousy always coincided with much unhappiness. Think back to your teenage days, when you were fond of a girl or boy, and how it hurt when this person spent too much time with someone else. It is only human that when somebody you love looks admiringly at someone else, jealousy creeps in. I especially say teenage days, because that is when we are at our most vulnerable. When we are secure in a relationship, it is more difficult for jealousy to take hold. So many people have failed to keep this jealousy in check, with the result that many lives have been ruined. At work we also see it, when for example one person is promoted ahead of another. Possibly the latter was even more capable in the eyes of others. It is always sad when jealousy, for whatever reason, takes over people's lives, as this undoubtedly leads to many problems.

I remember a female patient of mine of around forty who could not speak for crying. I soon discovered that she was overcome with jealousy. I prescribed heather, a flower essence in which I have great faith, because heather itself is a very jealous plant. Its jealous tendencies cause it to overgrow other plants. When this lady regained her speech she told me that she was absolutely convinced that her husband was having an affair with his secretary. She was by no means the first wife to suspect her husband, as employers who work closely with their secretaries sometimes mistakenly give the impression of closeness.

Although I eventually found out that she was very much mistaken about her husband's supposed infidelity, she had a jealous nature and mistrusted her husband as well as his secretary. The problems at home were getting out of hand to such an extent that neither husband nor wife could cope. In an effort to help her I prescribed some remedies and spoke with her at length, and fortunately in this instance the marriage was saved.

The parents of two teenagers told me that they were

having big problems with their eldest son. I learned that the parents had had to get married because she was expecting a baby, and because this had not been planned they went through a difficult time. The first child had somehow always lived with the idea that he was not wanted, just because he had not been planned. The boy grew up very jealous of his younger brother, which caused strain and difficulties at home. I advised the homoeopathic remedy Lachesis, which very much eased the situation. When attitude and behaviour become very difficult or awkward, I have also found the homoeo-pathic remedies Phosphorus and Staphisagra helpful. I have seen these help to keep the jealousy factor under control.

Neighbours who want to 'keep up with the Joneses' often act spitefully out of envy or jealousy. Their desire to have as much as the others – or, if possible, more – can lead to extremely unpleasant situations. In such instances I have found that Nux vomica or Sepia can be of help. Its effectiveness depends on the personality and character of the people involved.

Jealousy must be dealt with before it grows out of hand. In my work in British prisons I have met a great number of people who have landed in prison because of misdemeanours or crimes that were instigated by jealousy, and it is sad to see the price they have had to pay for this unfortunately very human trait. Not only do the criminals have to spend time locked up in prison, but their families also suffer greatly.

Often jealousy can block energy fields, and if the jealousy is deep-rooted and not recognised, it may be very difficult to unlock these energies. When a new baby is born into a family, an older child is often envious. In a young child this is often expressed in tantrums and rebelliousness, which should be acted on immediately. Holly or Emergency Essence, together with a great deal of understanding from the adults involved, will help to ease the situation. Never be afraid to show a child he or she is loved, and do not be fooled into thinking that the child is being difficult for the sake of it.

In cases of very severe jealousy that cannot be dealt with in any other way, the extract of sunflower – *Helianthus annuus* – may be beneficial, because it endorses the uniqueness of every individual. This may help to overcome deep-rooted jealous tendencies.

Who has not witnessed the jealousy of a girl who has lost her boyfriend to someone else? The girl becomes very jealous, her heart bleeds, and she must strive to overcome this emotion. The extract of the flower bleeding heart – *Dicentra formosa* – can often help to solve such a problem, while Dr Vogel's *Avena sativa* (twenty drops twice a day) has often been of great help in such situations.

A recent court case involving a man who had tried to murder his brother took my interest. Both brothers were quite religious, but one fared better in business and had a bigger house and a bigger car than the other. Presumably he was more capable or had a stronger personality. Why this was the case is not important, but sadly jealousy caused the less successful brother to attempt to murder the other. Fortunately the attempt failed, but the attempted murder case was tried in court and reported in the paper. From the courtroom report I understood that jealousy had been the motivation for the attempted murder, and it was jealousy that had affected the defendant mentally. This story so saddened me that, although I did not know the man, I sent him homoeopathic remedies, because I could not bear the thought of him going through life with this dreadful jealousy eating away at him.

We soon realise that this story is as old as mankind when we think of Genesis, the first book of the Bible. When God spoke to Cain after he had murdered his brother Abel, Cain answered, 'Am I my brother's keeper?' Indeed, we cannot possibly go through life without realising that we have the responsibility of being each other's keeper. After Cain had murdered his brother, he cannot possibly have enjoyed life because he would have been guilt-ridden. Unless jealousy is recognised and dealt with, there may be a very high price to pay.

Our destination in life is something we must learn to accept. It is painful to know that jealousy does not respect status. Even the life of a great leader such as the Israelite king Saul was ruined because of an uncontrollable jealousy. When the nation of Israel shouted 'Saul has slain thousands, but David has slain tens of thousands', something snapped within him. His jealousy cost him his life.

Learning to cope with jealousy or, better still, to overcome it, is a problem not only in the world of human beings but also in the animal kingdom. While I am writing this chapter I am looking out of the window over to the Clyde, and I can see thousands of little waves breaking on to the beach, in great harmony. It pains me to think how many lives have been affected by jealousy, disturbing the peace in one's heart, causing so many physical problems, because the three bodies were out of harmony. If I watch the little spiderweb on my window I see two small spiders who fight each other to get to the little fly that is caught in the web. It is a race to determine who will get there first, and I am sure that even in those little spiders' lives there is jealousy. If those feelings of jealousy could be controlled, the world would be a better place.

The opposite of jealousy is acceptance. My friend Dr Moolenburgh told me the story about two brothers. It is more a legend, with a great philosophy behind it. Long ago in the Middle East lived two brothers, who farmed adjoining sites. One of them was married with seven children, while the other brother lived alone. Each envied certain aspects of the other's life, while both of them felt embarrassed by this emotion. After the wheat harvest had been brought in, the unmarried brother could not sleep. Being on his own, the thought of having all that wheat somehow upset him, because his brother had eight more mouths to feed. He decided that he would give his brother some. This was his way to prove that he was stronger than his jealousy. He took two bags of wheat and in the night staggered to his brother's barn, where he left these bags. However, the married brother could not sleep either. He was concerned that his un-married brother had to go through life all on his own, and decided to give him some extra wheat to compen-sate for his loneliness. So in the middle of the night he went to his barn, selected two bags of wheat and delivered these to his brother's barn. Much to their asto-nishment, both brothers discovered the next morning that the amount of wheat in their barn had remained the same. Both wondered if they had only dreamt of having performed a good deed, so the following night they stayed awake and repeated this performance. Again the amount of wheat had not changed, so on the third night they took their bags and carefully made their way to each other's barn. It happened that where their properties joined, they ran into each other. They immediately understood what had happened, dropped their bags and fell into each other's arms, crying, 'Brother!' At that moment the Lord looked down from heaven and said that this was the place where He wanted a temple to be built. According to the legend, this happened on the place we now know as Jerusalem.

This complete and unconditional goodwill towards each other is the moral of the tale. The negative of this story is the well-known tale about two Russian friends, also farmers. Boris asked Ivan if he loved him. Ivan responded that as Boris had always been his friend, of course he loved him. Boris then asked, seeing as Ivan loved him, what was wrong with him. Ivan said he had no idea, at which Boris stated that Ivan could not possibly love him. We often come across this unwillingness to confide or to trust. Unconditional love is not a case of 'I'll scratch your back if you'll scratch mine'. The Greek word for unconditional love is agape, and it is this love that will help us to overcome jealousy so that we can accept the situation for what it is.

I witnessed the development of a sad situation when a man in his late thirties fell in love. The man had been very close to his mother, who had grown very possessive, especially since the death of her husband. The man was very happy, but the mother was not prepared to let go. She was viciously jealous and spoke to me about her jealousy. She actually admitted that she had done some awful things to try and drive the couple apart, and although I did what I could to help her, it was already too late. Her jealousy had gone so far that it had resulted in a very severe diabetic condition. A number of times she suffered a diabetic coma and the situation was very bad before I finally managed to persuade her to let go.

Unfortunately this is not such an unusual problem. I often see this with mothers who are very close to their children, more so than with fathers. My mother used to say that we only have our children 'on loan'. We may go through agony when they leave us, and I too struggled when my daughters left home to get married. Every time, I reminded myself of my mother's saying about our children being 'on loan', that we did not possess them. We may never claim them for life, as they have the right to live their own life. We should know when to let go.

Envy or jealousy sometimes creeps in and can do so much damage to a relationship. When help is necessary, I have used acupuncture treatment to balance the three energies of man. Let us be aware of the fact that we are individuals and as such are unique. This knowledge may make it possible to accept life and to accept the things that come across our paths, overcoming or avoiding jealousy that can so easily spoil our lives.

Chapter 4

DEATH ～ BIRTH

About a year ago I lost six friends in a relatively short period of time, six people who had been very influential in my life. Because of the quick succession in which these deaths took place, I spent much time pondering the finality and irreversibility of death. However, I also realise that one has no option but to learn to accept death. My closest mentor, Dr Alfred Vogel, was one of the friends I lost, and we last met one week before his death. During that last visit we reminisced and he looked back on a long life of many marvellous experiences, many of which I had shared with him over the last forty years. Although he was ninety-six years old he was still mentally alert, and he spoke of the many times we had gone to visit the gypsies in the mountains. We never failed to be impressed by their knowledge of herbs, plants and roots. I remember that on one of these trips Dr Vogel inadvertently trod on a plant, looked carefully at it and told me to take note of the way that the plant immediately recovered. His interpretation of this plant's characteristics was that the plant called out to be used in cases of trauma. This plant was arnica. The main characteristic, indeed, is that it helps people to recover from frights and shocks in the same way as it recovers quickly itself, just as it had bounced back when stepped on by Dr Vogel.

Dr Vogel and I recollected a number of our shared experiences. Some of them were laced with humour, some with sadness, but without doubt forty years of memories had bonded us into very great friends. Before I finally left him, I showed him a letter from one of the leading London hospitals inviting me to come and give evidence of a patient, diagnosed with an incurable disease, who was helped by the use of this natural medicine. Dr Vogel and I agreed that even this one instance was worth the pain in the past, when we had been criticised, misunderstood and sometimes ridiculed. Before I left we embraced, each with the knowledge that life is worth living – and even more so if it is dedicated to a worthwhile cause. When I use Dr Vogel's book *The Nature Doctor* for reference, I realise how fortunate we are to have such a rich reminder of him. In so many ways he expressed his belief in the importance of life, birth being a new beginning to fulfil the words of our Creator that life on this earth should be useful.

Another shock was when my dear friend Dr Leonard Allen died. Like Dr Vogel, he also functioned as a great mentor, and I am extremely grateful for the wealth of material he left me, some of which is even included in this book. We often spoke about life in general, and how best we could help people find better health. His long life was also one of total commitment to his fellow beings. I very often think of him because he left me all his books, as well as his research notes and material. Every day I see this collection of books in my library and I am more determined than ever to continue his work. Although life may not be perfect, we owe it to ourselves to make the very best of it under the circumstances.

Thereafter I lost my gardener, Peter, who had become a great friend. Often Peter and I shared many thoughts on organic gardening while we walked in the garden, usually early in the evening, inspecting the changes and making further plans. With every effort he could muster, he set out to prove that organic gardening could work. During one conversation I asked him why his leeks smelled so rich and his onions were so much bigger – why, in fact, all his produce was of such superior quality. His simple answer was that you only get out what you put in. What a pearl of wisdom, and how right he was.

Another good friend of mine, Linus Pauling, twice Nobel prize winner, died at the age of ninety-four. We had shared the stage on several lecture tours, and he had spent a lifetime helping others. Once Dr Vogel, Linus Pauling and I visited the Netherlands together. I was greatly impressed when he told us how, at the age of sixty-seven, he seriously considered retiring. Through some chance conversation he developed a sudden interest in vitamin C, and with a fellow countryman from Scotland, Dr Ewan Cameron, he set about researching the role it played in the treatment of cancer. Both put in a lot of work and Linus Pauling had a small book on vitamin C published, which changed his life. He did much for science throughout his life, and he said that in his 'other lifetime' he determined to share his knowledge with others and help them. This, to him, was the ultimate goal. He considered that from when he was sixty-seven years old until the age of ninety-four he had been granted another lifetime, and with vitality gained from a healthy way of life he could share his knowledge for the benefit of others.

Yet another friend was taken from us suddenly. I thought about the work that he had done, deciding to share his vision and make it available to others. With single-minded commitment, and at great expense, he set about establishing a clinic in the Netherlands, where a large number of people came to seek relief from pain. For a while we worked together in a clinic based in an area where the soil was rich in natural minerals, and he established a clinic founded on thermal baths. Unfortunately his life ended unexpectedly.

Last in this sequence of deaths, I lost my oldest patient, at the age of one hundred and eight. She had always led a simple but healthy life. She had borne thirteen children, so it was far from an easy life, but she had great stamina and determination. She was genuinely loved and respected, by her children, grandchildren and great-grandchildren as well as by her friends and neighbours. She had always agreed with me that one is as old as one's circulation and, as a blood circulatory remedy, she faithfully took St John's wort. At a later stage, to give extra support to her brain, I recommended that she should also take Ginkgo biloba (fifteen drops three times a day). This was her regime, and as she reached the age of a hundred and eight she could not have been far wrong in her beliefs.

All the people referred to reached a good age, although some obviously lived longer than others. It is sad, then, to think of how lives are lost before their time, many of them due to a general deterioration and erosion of the environment, threatening general health. This thought often depresses me, and I firmly believe that we have an obligation to respect, protect and nurture God's creation. By doing so we help to make the earth a better place to live, and we contribute towards a better life for all.

In a downhearted moment I suddenly remembered a promise I had made to God towards the end of the Second World War. We were fortunate that we lived to see the end of the war, and having met Linus Pauling I often remembered the little vitamin C tablets from the Red Cross. I have never doubted that we owed our lives to those little tablets. Since then I have been a great believer in the value of vitamin C, and I always bristle with indignation when the wisdom of taking vitamin C is called into question. Mostly this is done by people who do not fully appreciate the properties of the vitamin and how it undoubtedly saved my life. When I saw the destruction around Arnhem, where so many young lives were lost for so little gain, I promised God that if ever we were fortunate enough to survive the war, I would dedicate my life to helping people – and this is what I am still trying to do.

Death is not easy to accept, especially when it is a young person. From close by I have suffered with people who lost a loved one during the thirty years of civil unrest in Northern Ireland. Witnessing the destruc-tion of the lives of those who suffered the loss of a relative or a close friend, I have seen how cruel and far-reaching the effects can be. Yet we must learn to accept death, which is not an easy task, as we can only accept the unavoidable.

Only a few hours before he died, I spoke with one of my very best friends. He had totally dedicated his life to easing the plight of the poor and gave his life, under very difficult circumstances abroad, bringing some happiness into people's lives. When he was cruelly and abruptly taken from us, because of a progressive cancer, he accepted that as his fate. He departed from this life in the knowledge that he had done all he could, and was looking now for a better future.

In 1970 Elizabeth Kubler-Ross identified five stages through which a patient has to go when moving towards death. I must honestly say that those people I have been close to during the final stages of their life mostly seemed to accept the fact that death is an inherent part of life. Sometimes, however, we see a denial in the reaction of patients when they know their time is near. Secondly, the patient may become frustrated and angry. Thirdly, he or she may bargain with God or with the doctors. The fourth stage is when anger and bargaining have clearly not achieved the desired result, and depression can set in. Fifth and finally, although not all patients reach this stage, most then realise that there is nothing left but acceptance.

It is never more important to be able to communicate to family and friends than when preparing oneself for the end. Sometimes outside help is useful and a person who can provide spiritual guidance can bring solace and acceptance. This is not always required, however, because I have also seen people who accepted death and welcomed it as a victory. I saw this in the demise of my father, who was anxious to be taken because of his great suffering. From the way he had been brought up he knew about self-denial, and he suffered severe torture during the Second World War. He accepted that his life was at an end and went peacefully, in full spiritual acceptance. Once, when we spoke about the torture he underwent in those dark days during the war, he made a wise statement: it was not the physically strong who survived the concentration camps, but the spiritually strong, because they had more reason to live. This teaches us once more that the spiritual or emotional side of life is stronger than the physical part.

Communication is most important, and thankfully nowadays there is a focus on intervention, not only for the person who dies but also for those left behind. The three authors Lonsdale, Elver and Ballard in 1979 emphasised that humility and respect is better than flashy therapeutic skills, and the role of a comforter is as relevant as ever. After all, the end is the beginning.

I was impressed by the wisdom of a tale I read in a book written by I.V.M. Sweeney, a story of an old Chinese woman whose only son died. She visited a holy man to find out how to bring her child back to life. He said to her, 'Fetch me a mustard seed from a home that has never known sorrow and we will use it to drive out the sorrow from your life.' As she set off on her quest, her search for the seed was in vain. In the course of her journey, however, she found that she was not alone in her suffering. She heard tales of grief and sadness which abound in the lives of the rich as well as the poor and realised that bereavement is an inevitable part of life. The grieving mother found herself gradually drawn back into the business of living. Through the contact with others she regained her life.

Like the old Chinese woman, it is possible to sink so deeply into grief that it is hard to see a way out. Sympathy and understanding are very important, but not everyone is blessed with having trusted ones who can provide this. Remember, then, that medical relief can be provided, but I hasten to add that I do not believe in prescribing tranquillisers for this purpose, as this could easily result in a dependence on drugs. Ignatia is very often prescribed for coming to terms with grief. It is known to take the sting of death away and is a worthwhile natural remedy that helps people to overcome grief and accept death. Emergency Essence is also useful, as it contains some flowers that encourage mental healing. The extract of corn called *Zea mays* is believed to encourage a balance between heaven and earth, giving calmness when death is approaching. Monks, the healers in the past, often recommended chamomile (*Anthemis cotula*) because the flower was known to bring emotional peace. Today chamomile is still considered to be of help in such circumstances.

Other ways and means to overcome or accept grief and sorrow will be discussed in the next chapter.

The reverse of death is birth, and this phenomenon is of great comfort. Sometimes, when I again feel the loss of a particular friend, I make myself think of the many births that take place every day. These births constitute new life, with a lot of new opportunities. I then think of my own children and grandchildren, how happy they are and how, full of expectancy, they look forward to new opportunities. This realisation cannot fail to make one happy to know that one is still part of life.

One of my young grandchildren weighed no more than 1.8 kg at birth, and we hardly dared hope that she could hang on to life. However, that minute human being proved to have such tremendous will to live that it was of great encouragement to us all. As young and frail as she was, she showed sheer grit and determination to rid herself of the monitors, drains and equipment to which she was wired. She was fortunate because she had been blessed with good breathing and tremendous energy. It was this that allowed her to pull through, and it is with humility that I watch this child growing into a happy girl, and I thank God for His wonderful gift.

A new life encourages in us a protectiveness, and we want to take care of it. Newborn babies are given the best chance in life if the mother can breastfeed. In this way the baby's immune system is allowed to develop most fully. In my book *Pregnancy and Childbirth* I repeatedly stress the importance of a healthy food pattern, and few mothers would deny her newborn the best possible start in life. Young life needs proper nourishment and diet, and everyone wants to provide a healthy environment for the baby to flourish. It would not do to endanger that young life by withholding what is so important, such as fresh fruit and vegetables. When I think of the generations that have been raised under much more difficult circumstances, such as being born or growing up during the war years, I am forever grateful to my mother who gave me what she could by breastfeeding me for the first few months of my life. By doing so she provided me with the best possible start. This allows the immune system to benefit, which was especially important under those unfortunate circumstances I and many others experienced during our younger years.

A birth is nature at its best, and when one thinks of the perfection of the human body as mentioned in the first chapter, where skeleton, bones, muscles, nerves and mind combine into a human being, we thank God for His greatest gift imaginable. Birth is the positive side of death, and birth reminds us of great new beginnings. Up to the nineteenth century little was known about life. Now we know a little more, but with that knowledge we also know how much more there is yet to learn. We do know, however, that life is a constant renewal of cell tissue and that disease is a relentless breakdown. With that in mind we know how important it is to obey the laws of nature, and in doing so we will also obey the laws of God.

Chapter 5

GRIEF ～ SYMPATHY

The severe digestive problems of a middle-aged female patient were without doubt the result of the fact that this lady mourned the death of her husband, even though he had died more than twenty years ago. Her sorrow was part of her and it soon became clear that she had never come to terms with the loss of her husband. She had not been able to let go and she had actually never been able to stop grieving. Grief had affected her health, and what might have remained a fairly minor digestive problem had resulted in absorption problems. Her poor physical health was directly influenced by the fact that for the many years since she had lost her husband she had not shed a tear. This was not because she had not loved him, but because she had not been able to accept that fact. The grieving process had therefore never had the slightest chance of success, because it had never actually begun.

As this lady had never faced the fact that her husband

had died, she was emotionally unstable and at times suicidal. Because her husband had been taken away so suddenly, she had not been able to prepare herself for this loss. She had been devastated and bewildered, and in this frame of mind had not been able to come to terms with the loss and learn to accept it. Considering her deep emotional distress, it was actually surprising that she had managed to withstand the temptation to end her grief by committing suicide. It is always so much healthier if one can come to terms with the death of a loved one by allowing a period of mourning.

I was very touched when I heard her story, and the fact that she had not been able to grieve made me think of how our cultural background determines how we manage our emotions. In the different countries where I have lived, I have seen big differences in the ways people cope. In Scotland people tend to hide their feelings and put on a brave face. Generally one feels embarrassed about mourning or being in the presence of someone who mourns, and this characteristic is often a hindrance to the recovery process.

Not being able to express grief or sorrow over the loss of a person dear to you, whether it be through death or divorce, discourages the healing process and makes it all the more difficult to cope with the loss. This lady's story brought to mind the words of Shakespeare: 'Give sorrow words the grief that does not speak, whispers the o'erfraught heart and bids it break.' If only she had broken down and expressed her grief in a physical way by crying, she might have been able to learn to accept the loss. Contrary to the general belief in our Western culture, there is no shame in crying for the loss of a loved one. It might have helped her to gain strength from the love she had shared.

Unfortunately her health had been affected and the digestive problems had developed into a duodenal ulcer, which desperately needed treatment. I read somewhere that the journey of grief is sometimes difficult. The loss is the start, often followed by protest because of shock. Confusion is the next stage, searching the mind to determine what has happened, and unless a period of mourning is allowed the despair may turn into agony or depression. The usual sequence is that the moment will come to pick up the threads of life and try to get on as best we can. Sorrow or grief is easier to live through if it can be shared. The saying that 'company in distress makes smart less' contains much wisdom.

In Elizabeth Kubler-Ross's book *To Live Until We Say Goodbye*, we read that in battles with grief there is no better medicine that the showing of love and sympathy to a grieving person. Too often, especially with the loss of life in young children, I have witnessed that parents, having done everything possible, cannot come to terms with the situation, and that such a loss marks them for life. It is even more desperate when I see that their grief is such that their other children are emotionally neglected, which in turn causes emotional scars for them.

There are homoeopathic remedies that may relieve mental and emotional stress. Grief has its common features, but each individual experiences trauma in different ways. There is no right or wrong way to go through the mourning process. Remember, however, that every person who loses a loved one goes through the phases of acceptance and non-acceptance, and there is no harm in the shedding of tears. After a good cry one often feels better, although there is a certain numbness, as if nature applies a natural anaesthetic. These experiences are all part of the healing process of bereavement.

In the book *Death Belongs to Life*, the author states that a world without grief would be a world devoid of love. Indeed, if we are happy in a relationship, whether it be as parent, child or with a partner, it cannot fail to hurt when it is time to let go. Refusal to accept or guilt make it even more difficult to come to terms with a loss. When those in mourning pick up a photograph, a letter, a memento or a treasured possession of the person who has left, it may cause total recall of that person. Some people receive solace from this, while others will ban all such material from their lives. As I said, each individual experiences trauma in a unique way.

Words of sympathy should be carefully chosen, but they should not remain unsaid. There are many kinds of bereavement or grief, and there are different ways of living through such periods, but letting go is essential. It is said that grief is a fingerprint uniquely experienced by each person in relation to each separate loss. Everyone deserves to have a good listener for such moments of grief.

A trauma needs to be dealt with because we know that emotional sorrow can result in physical problems. Traumas are associated with a whole set of emotions, including fear, anger and lack of love, and there are homoeopathic remedies that can support us in overcoming grief without suppressing it. In homoeopathy we believe that a person's emotional condition is expressed through the body. In my experience, one of the best homoeopathic remedies to support and strengthen emotional stability in moments of grief is Ignatia, and sometimes I also prescribe Zincum valerianicum.

Although I have largely written about grief as the result of the loss of a loved one through death, the loss of a loved one through divorce is equally hard to accept, and the grieving that is associated with such a loss can be equally severe. Sometimes people find this even harder to come to terms with, because whereas death is not of one's own volition, divorce can leave one of the partners with a feeling not only of loss but also of inadequacy and rejection. I have often heard people in these circumstances express the opinion that it would have been easier to accept if the ensuing loneliness were indeed the result of loss of life. In such circumstances I recommend a flower essence called sticky monkey flower, the Latin name of which is *Mimulus aurantiacus*. This will help to relieve the terrible grief that is experienced when a partnership comes to an end. In some cases it is also good to give some Natrium mur.

The other day, an elderly lady who had lost her husband after a long and happy marriage confided that she was completely lost. In tears, she said that she needed a shoulder to cry on but that she had nobody who could fulfil that role. Often sympathy is all one can offer in times of grief. Sympathy can be shown by listening to the bereaved person, and sometimes a few words will be enough to help that person along the road to recovery and strengthen them in acceptance of their fate. Remember that it will do little or no good to say to a grieving person that they will have to pull themselves together and get on with life. Death is not easy to accept, but if you have loved and received love from someone, you must understand that one day it will come to an end.

I was told by a couple who were very much in love that the thought that something unforeseen might happen made them kiss each other goodbye every day as if it might be the last time. Personally I find this a rather morbid thought and I would find it hard to live that way. However, a certain wisdom is hidden in this idea, because we know that life does not last forever. This may be an irritating thought, but in some respects this attitude may make death a little easier to accept.

Furthermore, the feeling that one will be parted for only a little while provides people with a certain amount of comfort. Certainly this is a comfort to a religious person, but in modern times it seems that fewer people are able to embrace these views.

In lectures I remind my listeners that there are many therapies to help us overcome grief, for example osteopathy, homoeopathy, aromatherapy or reflexology, but sympathy is still the best of all. These forms of medicine need to be applied by a qualified practitioner, but sympathy can be given by a person from whom it is least expected. People who have experienced the sorrow and grief of a bereavement have learned how deep suffering can be and how bleak the outlook is without the loved one, and because they can speak from the heart, sympathy from another sufferer is of the greatest help. Remember that positive action and thought usually gives a positive result. Showing sympathy is a positive act, and therefore this provides most comfort to a mourner.

One of my younger patients, a beautiful girl whose

photograph I often look at, was diagnosed with brain cancer. With the help of natural remedies she lived longer than we had dared to hope and until the end she remained a brave fighter. Although she had accepted her fate, she was determined to live life to the full in the short time that was left to her. Three months before she died, she gave birth to a baby girl. At the moment she died, the baby in the cot stretched out her arms. We realised this was unintentional, but everyone present found it comforting.

One of my Dutch friends told me a story of overcoming grief which I found very touching. The headmaster of a small primary school lost his wife through illness and was left with a four-year-old daughter. They were devastated, and in their grief the father and daughter clung together. He felt that in this time of mourning he wanted to have her close to him, and although she had not reached school age he took her to school with him. The age of pupils in the primary class was around ten years, but this happened to be a class he was teaching. The little girl would sit very quietly during lessons in the class, safe in the knowledge that she was near her father. On a visit to the school a school inspector asked the girl what she was doing there. In a touching way, she answered that she was learning how to be still. I was suddenly reminded of this while writing this chapter, because we must learn to be still. Be calm, be still, and everything becomes new. We must accept death as we accept life, because the promise is there.

Chapter 6

LONELINESS ~ FRIENDSHIP

In the forty years that I have practised medicine I have come to the conclusion that loneliness is one of the worst diseases. I have met so many people who have in the privacy of my consulting-rooms told of their solitary struggles. I have learned to fear the effects of loneliness, and whenever I have recognised this tendency in my patients I have attempted to set aside time to try and get them to talk about themselves.

Many people are lonely, especially in today's society with everyone rushing around. Lonely people tend to shy away from others. It can be a very gradual retreat, comparable to a snail drawing back into its shell and shutting out the world. Perversely, the tendency of lonely people is to withdraw, instead of stepping out into the world and seeking company. Little do they realise that lack of communication and friendship may be detrimental to their health. Often I see illness that has been allowed to develop and fester because of loneliness, and quite often this is encouraged by the feelings of being misunderstood or feeling unloved. It is a hard world, and our material society is the reason that everyone seems to be rushing on to the next challenge or event. At the best of times it may be difficult to find a place in life, and if it is natural to withdraw or hold back because of some emotional block or embarrassment, shyness or lack of self-belief can result in ever-increasing loneliness. In order to receive, one must give, and in order to be accepted by others, one must accept oneself. Remember that sometimes it may require no more than an outstretched hand or a kind word to comfort someone in their loneliness.

When we moved into a new neighbourhood we were warned that our neighbour was an unpleasant woman and that she kept very much to herself. Apparently, she was a fervent photographer and the creator of some superb embroidery work. When I saw some samples of her work I was struck by the quality and I thought that anybody who could produce something so beautiful must be able to know a deeper sense of living. It was some time before I had a reason to go and see her and meet her as a neighbour. She asked me in because it was the polite thing to do, but she was by no means friendly. Hesitantly, a conversation developed, and I told her that I had seen some examples of her embroidery work and also her photography, which I very much admired. I suggested that she must live very close to nature. She responded by saying that nature was her only friend, as she had so often been disappointed in life. It soon became apparent that she had had a hard life and she mistrusted everybody. She had been disappointed so often in relationships that she had made up her mind not to allow anything like that to happen again, and therefore she lived a very withdrawn life. She would manage on her own, and by not involving herself with others, even her neighbours, she would not be disappointed again.

Sometimes it is easier to confide in an outsider, as there is a certain measure of safety in anonymity. You can unburden some of your emotions, safe in the knowledge that you may never have to speak to the person again. I don't know whether it was because she saw me in that role, but she told me that her husband had been a drunk, and her children had been a disappointment. One of her sons was in prison. She made no secret that life had not been particularly kind to her, and that she had no great expectations. Furthermore, her health was beginning to cause some concern. Through her actions and reactions, she had become a very lonely elderly lady.

I felt a great sympathy for this lonely person and pointed out that it was clear from the quality of her photography and embroidery work that she had good hands and eyes. She looked at me with an air of suspicion, yet she seemed to listen. At least she did not close the door to me. Slightly encouraged, I told her that it is within ourselves to bring some happiness, and in most cases sharing with others may indeed bring disappointments, but it will also reward us with friendship and understanding.

I have always greatly admired the work of the Samaritans and I had some involvement with them in the early years. When I carelessly dropped the name

'Samaritans' into the conversation, my neighbour immediately responded that she would have nothing to do
with them, because she was quite able to deal with her
own problems. I agreed, because she had a strong
personality, but thought it likely that she would need to
learn that the gift God had given her could be one way
of reaching out to people.

As time went by we became friends, and by gradually
getting involved in some community work, she made
friends who could see the lonely person behind an off-
hand exterior. I gave her a book which gives solace in
times of loneliness or distress, C.S. Lewis's *The Four
Loves: Affection, Eros, Friendship, Charity*. This has often
been a help to my patients, and I hoped it would help
my new friend. She developed into a charitable person,
and became able to cope with life's ups and downs. She
started communicating again with her children. Of
course, the change did not take place in a matter of
weeks, but the change was definitely there. That she
evolved into a different woman was not because of me,
but because it was within herself. She only needed
someone to reach out the hand of friendship, to bring
down her defences and to rekindle something in her that
had been lying dormant by the harsh experiences in her
life.

Too often I have come to the conclusion that loneliness may well be the worst affliction in this world. This
was also the case with a cancer patient who fought a
very lonely battle. She felt that nobody understood her
and nobody wanted her. Because the simmering cancer
was not progressive, she got little sympathy and understanding. In her loneliness she became self-centred and

was considered a nuisance, while all she wanted was some friendship and company in her lonely battle. In an effort to help her to contain her illness I prescribed an American remedy called Herbal Complex C, Petaforce from Dr Vogel and some vitamin, mineral and trace-element preparations. She responded well to these remedies together with a sensible diet, and she regained some balance in her life. I brought her into contact with some people who were similarly afflicted and, learning that they shared her experiences and disappointments, she came to accept her fate. This acceptance made her feel happier than she had been in her self-imposed isolation and she became a much happier person.

Loneliness is a negative emotion and therefore has a negative influence on our health. I can never over-emphasise how important it is that we respond in a positive manner if a lonely person looks to us for company or friendship. We cannot wash our hands of the situation by a negative response to the question 'Am I my brother's keeper?'. Indeed we are; we have a duty in life to help each other. I found that out with a pretty young girl who was diagnosed with incurable cancer. She was very embarrassed about her condition, and because her parents were no longer alive she had no one with whom to share her thoughts and concerns. Because of my profession she felt no embarrassment talking about her problems and therefore saw me as a person in whom she could confide. From her oncologist she knew that her life was drawing to an end. I also knew that was the case, and without raising her hopes for a recovery I tried to help her, giving her remedies to comfort her in her lonely battle. She often phoned when she was lonely, but at least there was somebody she could contact. During what turned out to be her last visit to the clinic, she thanked me for my help in easing her burden and said that she foresaw a happy future. She hugged me when we said goodbye, went home and died a day later. A neighbour who had kept an eye on her phoned to let me know that she had died. She assured me how meaningful and uplifting our friendship had been to this lonely lady. She had always looked forward to her visits to the clinic and our little chats had given her the strength to soldier on.

It brought home to me that loneliness is a very real problem for some people. I firmly believe that in our modern society loneliness is much more of a problem than it was for older generations. For example, often nowadays it is necessary for people to move away from their home area to find employment. This may leave elderly parents on their own, or, if the parent or parents move to be nearer their children, they leave their friends and all that is familiar behind.

We may flatter ourselves and think that we do not know any lonely people and therefore have no responsibility in this area. I can assure you, however, that if it is in our heart, we need not look far. Sometimes we meet elderly people whose lives are drawing to an end, and despite their memories of happiness they become lonely and need more attention. I witnessed exactly that with my own mother. She reached an age when she had lost most of her friends and she became lonely and introverted. She expressed a desire to join them, as life was lonely without their friendship. She was very disturbed when a long-time friend of hers committed suicide, the news of this death coming as a tremendous shock because she had never suspected that this friend could have been so lonely that she could be driven to this saddest of all deeds.

Contemplating the disastrous effects of loneliness reminds me of what I consider to be one of the failures in my professional career. It concerned a young woman who was severely depressed when I first saw her, and unfortunately I was unsuccessful, as I could not get through to her. Like her own doctor and minister I failed, as her own family had failed, to create a bond with her. I listened to the sad story about the man she loved and planned to marry, who had made promises, raised her hopes, and then abruptly broken off their relationship. The fact was that she actually did not want to be helped. She had convinced herself that she was beyond help and refused the helping hand I, and the others, reached out. She would not take the remedies I recommended. She was overcome with grief because this man, the love of her life, had let her down. She was one of the people I have seen dying of loneliness and a broken heart. There was nothing anyone could do to help this girl because she had nothing left to live for.

How different was the response of another girl who had been in a similar situation. She was let down in the same way, but on my advice took *Avena sativa* (twenty drops a day) and Ginsavita (one tablet twice a day) and responded very well. She slowly picked up the threads of her life again and positively tried to get over the fact that she had been rejected by a person with whom she had shared her life for ten years. Having shared her sorrow I was delighted when she told me what had happened when, on her way to a conference, her car had broken down. As she was parked on the hard shoulder of the motorway and trying to decide what to do, a sports car passed and, seeing her, the driver stopped and offered assistance. When her problems were solved, the young man who had helped her asked her out for dinner. In the knowledge that he had been there to help her when needed, she accepted his invitation. She told me that a friendship had developed that was so superior to anything she had known in her previous relationship that only now had she realised how foolish she had been to have mourned so deeply a relationship that had been so much less satisfying than what she had found now. She had found happiness.

Loneliness can manifest itself in many ways. As I write, I am looking at a photograph of a happy threesome, a woman with two young children. I met this lady a number of years ago when I was on tour in the USA. One day I was a guest in a huge health-food store. Despite the large size of this shop, it was so filled with people that one would think it was the last place to feel lonely. Yet this attractive young woman sat down, broke down in tears and told me how utterly lonely she felt. She told me that she had lost touch with her friends because they could no longer put up with her withdrawn attitude. Her husband was living his own life and no longer attempted to comfort her. She knew what was happening, but was unable to stop the further retreat within herself. The root of the problem was that she so desperately wanted to have a baby. So did her husband, but he contained his disappointment. She, however, felt increasingly dejected. Although there appeared to be no medical reason why she should not fall pregnant, her emotional anxiety caused her to keep others at a distance and draw further and further into herself. She feared that her husband blamed her for not being able to bear children and that before long she would lose him. As if the distress of her disappointment was not enough, the doubt about her marriage was further reason for depression.

I had very little material to work with in trying to help her. I browsed through the store looking for suitable remedies that might be of help. I selected a high concentration of vitamin E (600 IU twice a day), Dr Vogel's *Ginkgo biloba* (fifteen drops three times a day), three capsules of evening primrose before retiring at night, and half a teaspoon of wheatgerm oil. She left me in tears and in my heart I prayed that something would happen.

I did not see her again until I came back three years later on a visit to that same store. She walked towards me with two children and, looking very happy, threw herself into my arms and thanked me. Her parting words were 'I shall never forget the comfort and the friendship you offered in the hours when I felt most lonely'.

When I left the store that evening, after another very busy day, I was handed a letter, which I read later that evening in my hotel room.

Dear Jan de Vries,
My husband and I had been through ten years of endometriosis and infertility with every conventional treatment available, including three in-vitro

attempts. In February 1993 I saw you for ten minutes' consultation, where you gave me a prescription for ginkgo, vitamin E, evening primrose and wheatgerm oil. On the verge of another in-vitro attempt or adoption, we decided to follow your advice. I took the herbs for one month. On Mother's Day of 1993, to our total amazement, we had a positive pregnancy test. Our son was born in January 1994. On our son's first birthday we tried the prescription again for one month. Our daughter was born in October 1995. Since then, your 'recipe' has been responsible for three other babies, one due to be born this week.

You have changed the course of our lives. We are stunned and profoundly grateful.

People are very touched whenever we share our story. Have there ever been articles or medical studies written that can be shared with the medical establishment?

We wanted to write to you on our son's first birthday, and here you are in Oregon one week after our daughter's first birthday.

Thank you for making our children possible.

Friendship is wonderful. In the time of greatest sorrow it is good to find a hand of friendship. I wonder how King David felt when Jonathan, the son of Saul, reached out the hand of friendship and helped him avoid what could have been his death? When people in need see a hand of friendship, they will perceive this as positive support.

When people are dying, I have seen the positive effect

of having a friend who stands by them. Above all, many times I have seen gratitude when people have found a friend in Jesus when they battled in life's greatest struggle. This belief is of the greatest support to people when they meet loneliness on their journey through life.

In our suffering we can easily feel isolated, and friendship and affection is the best way to overcome this loneliness. According to ancient philosophers, friendship is the purest of all loves. In perfect friendship there is a love that goes beyond all other help that can be given. Unconditional friendship is often subconsciously given and is often difficult to express in words. It is not difficult to extend the hand of friendship to a friend, but it is very hard to show friendship to an enemy. We can, however, control our thoughts and our actions. Even with those we cannot see as friends, we must learn to value them for their good points. 'There is so much good in the worst of us and so much bad in the best of us that it behoves all of us not to talk about the rest of us.' This quote I found in a book I was given during one of my trips through the United States. Jim Farmer said, 'I have learned that to have a good friend is the purest of all God's gifts, for it is a love that has no exchange of payment.'

Remember that there is a great deal a lonely person can do for himself or herself. Find an interest in life, whether it be sports, relaxation exercises or a non-physical hobby. Such an interest will help to balance the energy positively, and in my book *Body Energy* I have written about this in much more detail. In times of loneliness it is possible to help oneself by creating positive energy.

So, if we come across loneliness, let's offer friendship by reaching out to the lonely, remembering that an outstretched hand can turn loneliness into friendship. When people suffer because of loneliness I often recommend St John's wort (Hypericum Complex), fifteen drops three times a day. A positive attitude develops because St John's wort beckons and pleads with us to recognise its message of love and friendship. St John's wort contains a message of love that can help us through life's worst struggles.

Chapter 7

GUILT ～ SELF-DENIAL

It is hard to believe the number of people I have met during my forty years in the medical profession who go through life with a guilt complex. Guilt is an enemy of oneself and guilt erodes a positive, happy attitude to life. We loosely use the term 'skeleton in the cupboard', but I believe there is no one who can categorically deny ever having done something of which he or she is ashamed. The problem arises when people cannot come to terms with this feeling of guilt. This can be done by atonement or confession, but it is up to the individual. If we cannot accept the benefit of forgiveness it can make our lives thoroughly miserable, and there are too many people who have not managed to find forgiveness or, more to the point, to forgive themselves, and who have ended their life prematurely because of this guilt complex.

I have met a number of people who have finally admitted to a guilt that has become part of their life. An elderly gentleman who lived a secluded and withdrawn life admitted in a self-critical moment that he had never found happiness because he had never come to terms with a wrong he had committed in his younger years. At the time we met the shame of this dark secret had had its effect on his health. I have said before that it is sometimes easier to confide in strangers, and he finally found the courage to unburden himself to me. He told me that quite some time ago he had been unfaithful to his wife. Because he had never told her, and therefore not been forgiven by her, he could not forgive himself. His own doctor had advised that it was unwise to upset his wife at this stage of their lives with a confession, as it was all in the past. This was something that she did not need to know, because it would upset her unnecessarily. Nevertheless, as he could not own up to this particular error, he could not find forgiveness himself.

With great honesty we discussed the situation, and as he was a religious person I told him that in self-denial he had the choice either to confess his fault to his wife or to pray and ask God for forgiveness. By admitting the guilt to his wife he might conceivably find peace within himself, but as his wife had not known about his infidelity he might burden her with a knowledge that would not be of benefit to anyone. He determined to make a clean breast of it and in his communications he confessed his guilt, and the feelings that had been with him for so long were lifted. Personally, I think that his first step in sharing it with me had been an encouragement to go further.

The senior partner of a law practice owned up to a misdemeanour that had haunted him all his adult life.

As he got older, the feeling of guilt that he carried with him was gradually destroying him. One of his very early clients in a new practice was an elderly lady who was entirely alone. At the start of his career as a young lawyer he had very little money, and he could not resist the temptation to take a little of her money, even though he knew that he was not entitled to it. He told himself that this extra money would help him to build up his practice. At the time, young and inexperienced, he felt that it was not dishonest to charge a little extra for the advice he had given her, because, after all, she had no one else and he had given her extra comfort by looking after her affairs. Little did he know at the time that later on in life the guilt over this dishonesty would become the one blot in an otherwise clean copybook. Since then he had always been honourable in his dealings with vulnerable people, but the shame of this one act preyed on him. Even though he was a practising Catholic, he dared not utter this admission even in the confessional, nor could he admit it to his wife. His shame and pride would not let him admit that error of judgement. As the elderly client had long since died, he could not find atonement by confessing to her.

The older he grew, the more this guilt reared its head, definitely affecting his health. That was how we met, and eventually he confided in me. I understood his dilemma, and in an effort to help him I told him a story that I once heard of a happening in a primary-school classroom. The subject of the lesson had been guilt, and the children fired several questions at the teacher. She then took a sheet of blank paper and with her pencil she made a mark in the middle. She showed the sheet of paper to the children and asked them to tell her what they saw. Every child, without exception, answered that they saw a black pencil mark. She compared this response with the subject of guilt. Why did none of the children see a white piece of paper?

There is a life full of goodness, a life full of helping others, spreading a loving, kind word – and then there is one black point. Something we have done in life that was not right. For a Christian it may be easy because that little black mark will be forgiven or erased by the forgiveness of God's son, who gave His own life to take away our sins. Very often people in life rely too heavily on this forgiveness. They harbour the comforting thought that now it is forgiven they need do no more about it. They should remember that there is still the point of self-denial, a process one has to go through to overcome the particular problem that bothers our conscience.

I told my friend that there was very little he could do, since the lady in question had died and he could not ask for forgiveness or return the money to her. What he could do, however, was to think of all the good he had done in life. He looked to me to be the kind of person who had lovingly helped people and sought atonement for his mistake. My suggestion was to take the sum of money and, with interest, donate it to cancer research, the Red Cross or the less privileged, to wipe the slate clean and rid his conscience of the guilt that had bothered him for so long.

In the Bible, King David committed the almost-unforgivable sin of having someone killed in order to please himself. In trying to atone, he looked for some-thing that could make him totally clean, and said, 'Wash

me with hyssop and I shall be whiter than snow.'
Hyssop has long been used as a cleanser and I advise
this remedy for people with high or low blood temperature caused by emotional problems. As the three bodies
of my lawyer patient – physical, mental and emotional –
were in distress, I prescribed hyssop (fifteen drops twice
a day). To help him to strengthen his nervous system he
took two Neuroforce tablets twice a day, and a capsule
of Stress-End. These remedies, in combination with his
method of atonement, brought him peace of mind.

Energy exists in spirit as consciousness, in mind as
thoughts and in emotion as feelings. A guilt-ridden person will experience a disturbance in his energy, as guilt
disturbs one's spirit. Our body is one great force field.
We can think of different names for it, such as electricity,
gravitation, light, sound, heat or colour, but basically
these are different forms of energy. The energy field of
the body can be disturbed by anything that preys on our
mind. In today's society there are many threats to this
energy field: the air we breathe, the food we eat, the
people we know, our thoughts and feelings. The environment in which we live is fundamentally concentrated
in an energy field that radiates and absorbs frequencies
and waves of energy. The waves are so minimal and so
vibratory that our senses are very often dimmed with
the right outlook to positive life. We are unaware of
these little energy waves or vibrations that do exist and
magnify a field composed of energy.

If we place a magnet under a sheet of cardboard, iron
particles sprinkled on to the cardboard will align themselves in the patterns around the magnet. Scientists call
these the lines of magnetic force. If we look at how

quickly this force can be disturbed by thought alone, we may better understand how guilt may be upsetting the energy field of the body. Our health is influenced by the function of the subtle energy fields that operate in and around the body. In advanced thinking, we look at the scientific aspects of it and the energy field in the spirit of the body manifests itself as an awareness, a consciousness or an intent or will. This we saw in the case of my lawyer friend. Spiritually he was in a turmoil because his guilty conscience affected the mental body which is composed of attitudes, ideas, beliefs, thoughts and a record of all experiences. Then our emotional body is composed of feelings, sensations and desires. Our physical body, as the result of all bodies, is composed of chemicals and tissue. The whole system of energy communicates between the various bodies where energy corresponds with our neuroplexus, our endocrine glands, our meridians and our energy within.

All individuals have different patterns of energy, vibrations and tones and they tune into life according to their individual character. If you strike a note on a piano keyboard, you get a sound and simple vibration. The hitting of a second note is the beginning of a harmonic sound. Emotions such as guilt will result in illness or disease. To restore harmony it is therefore important that something is done to restore those energies physically, mentally and emotionally.

The reverse of guilt is self-denial. The thing I hated most in my younger days was having to deliver things to people's homes. At home we had a pharmacy and if a patient or a doctor urgently required medicine, I had to get on my bike and deliver the goods as quickly as possible. Sometimes this had to be done in the middle of the night and in all kinds of weather. I had been instructed by my parents that after having rung the doorbell I had to take off my hat, stuff it under my arm and wait for the door to be answered. I had to look the person who opened the door in the eye and not lose eye contact until the door was closed again. I hated this job because I always felt embarrassed, but nevertheless it instilled in me the idea of giving something of myself to a person I did not know.

Another way in which my mother and father were very strict about self-denial was that I had to learn to ask to be pardoned or to apologise if I had overlooked anything or done anything wrong. They believed that if you did something for which you ought to be sorry, a self-denial should take place and you had to admit your wrong. My mother often told me that the lowest place is always open, it is never occupied, so I should take that place. My parents probably saw that as a child there was a form of self-righteousness in me that should be stamped out the hard way. Although it was not always easy, it was something that I have been very conscious of all my life. In life there are situations when it is especially difficult to give in or where self-denial goes against one's nature. Then this act of self-denial proves a strength of character. I admit that there were times when I felt that I was right, yet I was taught to adopt self-denial to make myself stronger – which is not an easy thing to do.

I have done a lot of work in British prisons, where I have met people who, I know, were influenced by circumstances to do the wrong thing. In several cases I have been able to help them come to terms with their guilt by bringing them in touch with the injured party. This worked beneficially for both the injured and the guilty party, because the confession of guilt worked as a catalyst for healing for all involved. Sometimes such action also helped the authorities to decide that the prisoner could be released earlier. Life is all about giving and taking. Dialogue and understanding sometimes makes self-denial and atonement possible.

I am not saying that self-denial is always easy; far from it. In this world many stand on their rights, but we must ask ourselves if it is healthy to become hard and bitter. Remember that the old Book says that 'bitterness can become the rotting of bones', and never a truer word was spoken. As a wise saying goes, life catches up with us and teaches us to love and forgive each other. William James (1842–1910) stated that the greatest discovery of his generation was that a human being can alter his life by altering his attitude of mind.

A female patient sought my advice after having consulted numerous practitioners about her constant headache. It was not difficult to see that she suffered greatly, but there appeared to be no physical reason for these headaches. In conversation I soon discovered that she had a guilt complex and was desperately seeking a way of solving that guilt problem. She was so headstrong that she suffered these headaches rather than using self-denial. Finally I managed to convince her that self-denial was essential, and fortunately, after admitting her guilt, her apology was accepted in love and she became good friends with the person she had so badly maligned in the first place. Her headache problem was solved.

Chapter 8

⊙

HATE ∼ LOVE

The other day I found a patient sitting in my consulting-rooms who vehemently stated that he hated his wife. He said that he could stand her no longer and that she drove him to distraction, and his emotions frightened him because he was scared that this hatred could make him do something he might regret. He was at his wits' end because of hatred for his wife.

Hate has brought many people to an untimely end, and it is probably one of the world's worst enemies. Some time ago I experienced a despicable form of hatred between two people who could drink each other's blood, as it is commonly expressed. Although this event happened in Northern Ireland, it was not related to the well-known problems between Catholics and Protestants. It concerned a hatred between two individuals that made them destroy each other's property. It is so sad to see how far hatred can drive people apart, people who ought to be living alongside each other peacefully. War, crises, lack of understanding and wrong communications can all cause a hatred that is very difficult to overcome unless one can talk to the other party. It is senseless to allow such hate to fester and ruin lives.

Hatred is often born out of jealousy, perhaps because the other party has something you don't have, but want. It may be because the other person gets promoted, and you don't. The other may be more gifted, and you feel inferior. When does dislike turn into hatred? When does hatred grow out of control? Hatred can influence even strong characters and drive people to commit deeds of which they would never have considered themselves capable. Hatred can lead to the ultimate crime of murder. I come back to the hatred between King Saul and King David. The underlying reason why Saul hated David was jealousy. It was this jealousy that drove him to such hatred that he felt like killing David. Because of the love of David, basically his love for God, who had anointed Saul as king, David stood back. Yet that great hatred in Saul's heart instilled by jealousy brought him to self-destruction.

I have had patients lose their self-control when they speak to me about hatred, and the resulting physical and mental destruction exacting its toll on their health is clear to see. There was the case of an elderly gentleman, the organist in his church, whose son had murdered the man's wife. Surely he could be forgiven for the hatred he felt towards this son? This man's health had been so badly affected that nearly every week he needed manipulative treatment of the spine to keep him straight, as every bone in his body was affected by his mental stress.

Unknown to him, while in prison his son studied to become a minister in the church. Because he had not been aware of this change of direction in his son's life, it came as an even bigger shock when he heard of the appointment of his son as the new minister in the church where he played the organ. This was a dreadful experience and he was completely distraught when he came to me. We talked at length and I carefully pointed out that his son must have changed a lot in order to change the direction of his life so drastically. His hatred for his son made that difficult for him to accept. He admitted that even the thought of having to play the organ during a service led by his son, bearing in mind that he had killed his mother, was abhorrent to him. I then told him that as it must be assumed that his son had been forgiven by God, his father should also forgive him and love his son. He thought deeply about this, but the time was not yet ripe. The happy outcome was that eventually they met in the course of their duties and in time there was forgiveness and an acceptance between them. Hate can sow the seeds of self-destruction that can never be cleared if one does not accept that positive love can overcome hatred. As a child I saw some awful deeds during the Second World War, and through life I have seen much hatred, but I am happy to say that hatred, when replaced by positive love, can be reversed.

How to overcome hate? Is there a way for man to overcome hate, and, if so, how can that hate be replaced by a positive love? I was very encouraged by a story I heard from my good friend Dr Hans Moolenburgh. In Haarlem, the Dutch city where he lived, a watchmaker and his family during the war gave shelter to some persecuted Jews. In the end they were betrayed and two sisters, Corrie and Betsy, were deported to the concentration camp in Ravensbruck. Largely due to the treatment of a very cruel female guard, Betsy died. Corrie miraculously survived the war, and later gave a series of lectures on her experiences. One day, after a lecture in Germany, she was approached by a woman who admitted that she had done terrible things during the war but said that recently she had become a Christian and was seeking forgiveness for her deeds. She told Corrie that she had agreed with God that she would not be forgiven until one of her former prisoners forgave her personally. She then asked Corrie for her forgiveness.

She had been recognised by Corrie as the cruel guard who had been responsible for the death of her sister. Corrie stood rooted to the ground and realised that she did not have it in her to forgive this hated woman. Then she remembered the line from the Lord's Prayer: 'Forgive us our trespasses as we forgive those who trespass against us.' Our sins cannot be forgiven if we do not forgive other people. So, not because she felt forgiveness, but because she obeyed the scripture, she put out her hand and forgave the woman. Only after she had acted in that way was she flushed with real compassion for that woman. Love is something we all need, and in this loving act of Corrie's she received greater love in her life and was a great blessing to others.

We also find this in our work. Healing is closely related to love but we should never believe that a doctor or practitioner heals or cures. They are only the tool, because only God heals. If we have His blessing, we can see what we have to do and the part we have to play. It is wonderful that in love we can overcome a hatred that may burn in our heart and eventually destroy us.

If we look at the world today, we cannot fail to want to find a solution to all this hatred and destruction. It is only through love that we can look at this world positively and it is only through love that we can save this world from destruction. Man has done much to destroy the beauty of nature and from this destruction many health problems have ensued. Happiness has been taken away because of the unloving and cold attitudes where money and greed have taken over so much of the power in this world. Yet love can cure hate.

Chapter 9

FEAR ~ COMMUNICATION

My father often said that fear is man's worst enemy. In the course of our work we find that a person's life can be ruled by fear – fear of the unknown, fear for oneself, or fear for the sake of fear. In one of my clinics I saw a lady in the waiting-room, shivering and visibly distraught. I asked her what was wrong and she replied that she feared the worst, but could not possibly talk about it. Later I learned that she had had some dreadful experiences in her life, which had left their mark. The ever-present fear in her life was that she might have cancer, and this was the overriding concern that never left her and took away any pleasure that she might have found in her life. Every waking moment was devoted to thinking about what she would do if cancer were to take over.

In an attempt to make her see things realistically I told her that she had no reason to believe that she had cancer. I pointed out that although she displayed no sign of cancer, a cancer cell is like a brain cell, and therefore could be influenced positively or negatively. To put it in a nutshell, cancer cells are cells that are out of control, often being called rogue cells. A constant negative influence may actually induce suspect cells to go out of control, as the mind is stronger than the body. I had managed to get her attention and she listened closely when I continued to tell her that there are positive cells and negative cells, or cells of regeneration and cells of degeneration. If the cells of degeneration become too many or too powerful, then there is a problem. Mentally, physically and emotionally, by harbouring the fear of cancer, she was asking for trouble. From her reaction I realised that she understood the message. I told her that I had known people who, because of a fear for their future health, changed their lives immediately, and with the aid of visualisation techniques they were successful in overcoming this fear which had almost become a way of life to them.

Having said that fear is one's worst enemy, I hasten to add that there are positive as well as negative fears. Crossing the road and being afraid of the traffic, thus making sure you are aware of the traffic and cross at the right time, is only positive. But fearing and imagining the worst will often bring trouble.

Energy blockages because of fear can lead to a change in personality. Shyness, anxiety, phobias, fear of the future, of accidents, of poor health, of spiders or insects, all kinds of hypersensitivities, fear of flying, of loneliness and many more anxieties can mar life. Usually with any of these fears I advise people to take Emergency Essence, composed of flower essences, while another wonderful remedy for fear is *Ginkgo biloba*, which also helps negative fears.

I sometimes tell patients who have a problem with fear to look at the sunflower – *Helianthus annuus*. Looking at the sunflower one gets a feeling of overcoming fear, and I am happy that cancer groups use the sunflower as their symbol because it expresses individuality and a uniqueness and healing relationship with one's Creator.

In another country I have a girl under treatment who is possibly the most attractive girl I have ever seen, but her life is filled with fear. Her upbringing was very distorted, and she received very little love from either her father or her mother. She was afraid of everything imaginable and unfortunately these unspecified fears eventually drove her to drink. This addiction caused a lack of appetite and she became anorexic and went from bad to worse. When she finally came to see me she was a shell of a person, a bundle of suicidal misery, and a great deal of talking was required to reframe her mind. With the help of a psychologist, and a lot of patience, we slowly got her on to the right path and turned her away from certain self-destruction. She learned to talk freely about the fear that had come into her life when her mother died when she was aged ten. Her father was always busy and totally incapable of loving this young and impressionable child. She reacted very well to Sunflower Essence and Dr Vogel's Centaurium (fifteen drops twice daily), and because she was in need of certain nutrients I prescribed zinc, which is usually of great help to anorexics. At various stages of her treatment I also prescribed Ginsavita, vitamin C and some multi-vitamin preparations. With the further help of acupuncture treatment she overcame her drink and drugs problem, and she learned to take her place in life. I am convinced that what made her turn the corner was the realisation of the destructive influence of her fears, and through frequent consultations with the psychologist and myself she came to realise how good life could be.

In my book *Stress and Nervous Disorders* I wrote that whilst love is our natural inheritance, fear is something the mind invents. In other words, fear is generated in the mind. Often when things are not going well and we are up against problems, there is a temptation to look at what is going to happen in the future, and unless we have a positive approach, we invite serious problems.

This case reminds me of another female patient who was in a similar situation. She was so overcome with worry about existing and non-existing problems that she could no longer cope. Then a 'friend' introduced her to drugs. She went from bad to worse, and when she came to me she was frightened of her own shadow and had lost any hope or expectancy for the future. By that time she was like a little bird, with very little body weight left. I will never forget what she told me: 'Everywhere I go I take myself with me, and the fear that is with me all the time makes me so scared of myself that incidents follow me everywhere.' In other words, she was asking for trouble, but at least she was beginning to realise that she was the one who invited these problems. I felt slightly encouraged to learn this and felt that there was some hope if she knew that most of her problems were based on fear and were therefore self-imposed. After treatment to wean her from her drug addiction, she also learned to conquer her fears. She gradually began to rediscover some pleasures in life and I am so pleased to say that she now does a lot of good work by sharing her experiences with others. She is involved in a number of self-help groups and is able to encourage others who are in a similar situation. This is yet another example of fear being overcome by communication.

In the previous chapter we mentioned that loneliness is one of the principal causes of depression. We often find that this is rooted in a failure to communicate. I sometimes look at people who have lost their sense of purpose in life, people who can no longer communicate and people who, when fear or anxieties have taken over their lives, wonder what has gone wrong. What was it that prompted them to turn their back on society? There are many contradictions in human society, science and technology. Although they have brought people together, they have also caused a gap in communication with each other. Man is basically a social animal and without co-operating with others there is little for him to enjoy. Real communication has its relationship in the day-to-day living at home or at work. Words are not always required, because a hand movement or a look can communicate between two people a sense of friendship, or indicate support for an individual if that is required at that moment. This is the kind of communication we often see between a mother and a child. This unconditional communication can help a child to overcome fears, because it feels close to the mother. Good communication results in strong and reliable relationships. I sometimes wonder what is the future of the world if we no longer communicate on a personal level. People who are full of anxieties are often so withdrawn within themselves that they forget the importance of communicating their fears or anxieties with others.

Mental approach and attitude are very important for successful communication. Learn to approach others positively, overcoming an inner conflict. Positive fear can be protective as long as we deal with it in a positive way by communicating the problem to others, and subconsciously there is much we can do with a communicative attitude. Positive thoughts place expectations around the corner, while negative thoughts will show up right in front of you. Harriet Beecher Stowe wrote, 'Point to ponder tomorrow – you're getting ahead of yourself now.' Slow down, savour the moment. When you get into a tight place and everything goes against you, never give up, for then and there is just the time and place that the tide will turn. If you want to, you will find someone there to help you. Always remember that fear can be overcome through love and communication.

Chapter 10

SADNESS ~ HAPPINESS

A middle-aged gentleman told me how sad he was, without going into details. When I had asked him several times why he was so sad, he reluctantly told me that he had made a great mistake. He had overstretched himself in business and through poor judgement he had lost a lot of money in a particular venture. His health was suffering and he wanted help to overcome the resultant stress and anxiety. In the telling of his story I heard him repeat several times how sad he was. He happily accepted my suggested treatment method of acupuncture and osteopathic manipulation to release these feelings of sadness. I pointed out, however, that I could not give him happiness, because that was only his to achieve. In a man-to-man talk I emphasised that he should count his blessings. He was not bankrupt, he still had his house and his car and, moreover, he still had the love and support of his family. There was no reason why he should not set out to make up for what he had lost, especially now that he was wiser because of his experience. He saw the point but nevertheless showed no signs of cheering up during the next three or four visits to the clinic. Then one day I saw him in great form, and he proudly told me that he had closed a marvellous deal which had made him a handsome profit.

This is a simple story but nevertheless it made me think how little things can influence our lives to make us sad. Sadness is not without reason, but we often see that sadness is brought upon us by ourselves. In this case, the man's unhappiness was dictated by the material success in his life. To me, that is a sad state of affairs.

A friend of mine once told me that we should see life as a big shoe shop, with shelves crammed full of shoe-boxes. She said that all those boxes in our mind contain experiences we have had, be they sad or happy. If we open a shoebox and find a pair of shoes of sadness, we take another box from the shelf and try on a pair of shoes of happiness. This is easily said, but it is undoubtedly a good philosophy. When there is sadness, it can be overcome by looking back and remembering happy times and concentrating on one particular area.

A while ago a patient of mine lost his wife. He was terribly upset about his loss, but I gently pointed out that he ought to remember how they had celebrated their golden wedding. They had both told me of the wonderful time they had had. Now he should think of all the people who would never have the opportunity of celebrating their fiftieth wedding anniversary. His face lit up, and the thought obviously brought him comfort.

Life is like a garden which brings forth weeds, flowers and vegetables, produce that can either be useful or useless. There is sadness and there is happiness, and undoubtedly the fruits of happiness will be greater than the fruits of sadness.

Happiness is a great remedy. Something mysterious happens in our body when happiness takes over. The tension breaks and the millions of muscle fibres seem to work in better co-ordination. The nervous system is controlled by the cerebrum, which is influenced by the will. Happiness is self-perpetuating.

As a diabetic, I know that I have a tendency to suffer slight depression or sadness about life. The other day, after I had spent a long and tiring day in the clinic, seeing so many problems, I felt inexplicably sad until I picked up a letter from a person who had written to me about a great sadness. Her son had been shot during the troubled times in Northern Ireland. She said that her sadness also brought happiness for the comfort, the friendship and the love she had received from others. Any time she felt sad, her happiness at finding so many new friends and so much love helped her through. Her courage and optimism were enviable, and my sadness disappeared like snow under the sun.

If happiness is important for the soul, it is also very important for the liver. I often explain at lectures that the liver influences our mood. The liver needs happiness, and diabetics with a tendency towards sadness should know that the inner secretions of the islets of Langerhans will increase production of insulin and sugar in the blood for better oxidation. A healthy attitude to diet is so important for a diabetic.

Often, people who experience sudden moments of sadness will be greatly helped by Milk Thistle Complex.

This is a remedy designed by Dr Vogel to help in the cleansing of the liver – and when the liver works well, one feels happier. We often see that some of the emotions we have discussed, such as envy and jealousy, are very powerful enemies, capable of destroying happiness. Our health will benefit if we strive for happiness.

I remember one of Dr Vogel's stories about an Indian prince who marvelled at one of his fellow believers, a poor man who could rejoice without envy at the beauty and gracefulness of the prince's wife. The puzzled prince questioned him, and the poor man explained happily, 'Why should I not rejoice in beauty, especially if it does not involve any worry or responsibility on my part? You have the burden of overseeing all your wealth and of providing for all your wife's needs, while I on the other hand can rejoice by just looking at her without any worry or dismay.' Very often in life we see that happiness is taken away by the opportunities that pass us by. If we look at life and at what is given and entrusted to us, and if we look at the treasure of nature, we can rejoice and be grateful for all that life brings.

We are fortunate if we can go to sleep and wake up with happy thoughts and if we can joyfully apply ourselves to our work and our duty. To bring happiness to people who are ill or wounded physically, mentally or emotionally is the best we can do. Happiness can transform life for someone who is sad and depressed.

In a little book on relationships, given to me after a lecture in Toronto, I read the following: 'Happiness is good. The place to be happy is here. The time to be happy is now. The way to be happy is to help make others happy.'

Chapter 11

OBSESSION ~ COMMON SENSE

In previous chapters I have mentioned that negative thoughts can lead to obsessions of many kinds. An obsession, albeit small in the first instance, can develop into a major problem, and as such it can grow so big that it can rule our lives. There are many forms of obsession. During typical uncertainties that are part of growing up, many children are obsessed about being too small or too big, being too fat or too thin, being shy, or not being physically attractive. Obsessions can be many, but worst of all is the realisation that one has become obsessed about certain things that cannot be changed. The time has come to realise that these characteristics can only be approached by common sense.

After a long chat with a young girl I eventually discovered why she had become anorexic. Her anorexia resulted not out of an obsession about her body weight, but because she felt that her ears were sticking out. In her mind this problem took on such major proportions that she withdrew into herself and became lonely, and the obsession led to a severe case of anorexia nervosa. I asked her why she was not bothered about her anorexia, because her face now looked so thin and emaciated that her ears seemed to be sticking out even more. As it is very difficult to get through to an anorexic, I first spoke with her about her background and her school years before I broached her anorexic condition. All the time I reassured her that she need not be worried that I would try to make her fat, as I know that, contrary to popular belief, fat people are rarely happy with themselves. I gently pointed out that because she was losing so much muscle she was slowly dwindling away. She responded well and listened carefully when I told her that if she really wished it, something could be done about her ears. At the present stage, however, her main concern should be her face, as well as her waist, instead of her obsession with her ears.

Obsession is a disorder, categorised by the presence of recurrent ideas and fantasies. Repetitive compulsions and actions can often lead to an obsessive compulsive disorder or an obsessive neurosis. Often anxiety is at the root, and treatment for obsession can be very time-consuming. A patient with an obsession can no longer think rationally and usually has a distorted vision of the specific problem that he or she has become obsessed with. A compulsion, although close to an obsession, is a more autonomous, characterised problem, but very often the overwhelming idea or image linked to obsession grows into an anxiety stage where realistic thinking is no longer possible. This can lead to a neurotic problem that is more difficult still to treat. I often feel that not only do patients with an obsession require compassionate understanding, a psychologist or a psychiatrist is also absolutely essential.

The other day I saw a young man who was obsessed about religion. He dreamed of going out and preaching the gospel as a modern-day missionary, but his religious leaders rejected him as unsuitable for this purpose. I could see their point, as he was not a balanced man and I could see that the stress of such a task would be too harsh on him. However, he felt that as he was being called, why should others object and why shouldn't he have the chance to show his worth? He felt obsessed with the idea that he was not considered good enough, and this obsession caused a nervous breakdown. He was in great need of guidance and counselling.

Tiber syrup, a French syrup mainly derived from herbs, and the nerve tablet JayVee from Nature's Best (two tablets twice a day) are very helpful for obsession. These remedies usually calm the nervous and are therefore ideally suited for someone with an obsessive nature. For obsessive compulsive disorders, electro acupuncture is of help, and sometimes manipulation will release stress, as often obsessions stem from stress situations. The obsessive patient should first of all learn to relax and face the problem. It is possible for obsession to develop into a hysterical or neurotic condition if the patient is not given the required help. Talking and listening are as much help as remedies in such conditions, and it is necessary to deal with such problems before it is too late.

Joanne, a very nice young girl, was so obsessed about

her weight that she became a typical victim. When we first met she immediately blurted out that she was unattractive because of her size. This was definitely not the case, but she had lost all sense of reality. I told her that her problem could be overcome, but she was so far gone that she had already become neurotic and had been rejected by her family as emotionally unstable because they could not cope with her. She went completely off the rails and, because of the embedded belief that she was fat and unattractive, she gave herself to any man who showed the slightest interest. On her return from a holiday that was spent once again in proving to herself that despite her weight she was still attractive to men, she lived in great fear that because of her low morals she might have contracted AIDS. Her obsession spiralled further out of control. She was a bundle of nerves and well on the road to self-destruction. We had to start right at the beginning, but fortunately she is slowly coming to the conclusion that common sense prevails. I have not yet given up hope that she may return entirely to her previous good health.

I often use the saying 'there is nothing common about common sense'. How difficult it is when one has lost common sense and is no longer able to recognise reality. When common sense is lost, everything is lost. Concerning destiny, Lao Russel said, 'He who would command his destiny must first learn how to balance the conditions which control it. The control of life is very often lost when the knowledge and the desire to steer one's own life is lost. He who has knowledge and desire may steer the ship of life anywhere he will, but he with little knowledge and desire is not even aware that he has a rudder with which to steer the ship of life.'

It was Joanne's own doing that wrecked her life physically, mentally and emotionally. She had to bring harmony back into her life, and in order to do so we had to start at the beginning. Every man determines his own destiny by his thoughts and actions every moment of his life. You can become what you want to if you are true to your thoughts and actions, but the measure of your desire must be great in order for you to become great. No one who has ever reached great heights has done so alone. We can see that the greatest men in the world are those who are the most humble.

I saw this with a young man who dearly wanted to go into the police force but could not do so because he had a speech impediment. He stuttered and fell over his own words, which became an obsession for him. I gave him acupuncture and impressed on him that he should try and speak more slowly. His common sense told him that he should try and follow my advice. The stutter was a problem that became a vicious circle, in that he started to stutter because he was worried that he would not find the words or make himself understood. We tackled the problem together, and with some remedies providing him with extra help, he actually cured himself by applying common sense to his problem.

Common sense is a wonderful expression. It is one of the most important parts of life, to be able to sit down and consider a problem that potentially could develop into a major concern or obsession. One should never lose sight of the fact that with common sense, most problems can be overcome. Common sense has an extra sense of solving power.

Chapter 12

STRESS/TENSION ~ RELAXATION

Stress, without doubt, is a very 'in' word these days. Everything seems to be related to stress, and when I recently visited arguably one of the best scientists in the world, I observed that physically he was under par. We talked about the stresses of life and came to the conclusion that stress and fatigue are two entirely different things. Often stress is caused by any one of four factors: improper food, improper temperature, improper rest and improper elimination, and sometimes by a combination of these. He said that an imbalance of these four factors was detrimental to health, and I could see what he meant. Somehow people under stress tend to eat high-protein meals, which is wrong, as they should be on a low-stress diet, balancing the carbo-hydrate with the protein intake. As far as temperature is concerned, I agree that in a country like Great Britain the temperature is not always conducive to relaxation.

Proper rest is too often taken for granted, but the quality of restful periods and relaxation is vitally important to counter the demands of stress. Healthy elimination, too, is often underestimated, and we should take this into consideration when we decide what to eat and drink. Healthy elimination means that waste material is not allowed to build up with the onset of stress into what is recognised as one of the most telling signs of a stressful situation: irritable bowel syndrome.

What happens with stress? When the body becomes stressed there is the dangerous development of a break-down, distortion or destruction of joints, bones or muscles. I often see that stress influences bones, muscles and nerves, encouraging a condition that causes a toxicity of the body. Stress undoubtedly also causes an imbalance in the alkaline-acid system. We often see that an acid body is affected by stress, causing duodenal, peptic or gastric ulcers, arthritic conditions, eczema, psoriasis and other related diseases. In such instances we must not only strive to reduce stress, we must also adopt an acid-free diet to overcome these problems.

My friendly scientist said that gravity was the underlying cause. Tensions, because of today's lifestyle, become stressful, and this places the body under threat. The nervous system works like the battery of a car in that it has a plus and a minus. If the battery runs low, it should not be charged with high-protein food. A balanced food pattern is needed to provide energy for the battery.

It is interesting to see how the body is made and how this human machine works. Firstly we have the skeleton of bones, held together by ligaments, to provide control of the joints by nerves. Secondly there is the mind, and thirdly there is that extremely delicate processing and manufacturing plant which is contained in the body and usually designated as the viscera. The raw materials we eat are converted into products for the various components. These three parts, while often viewed separately, are actually one functional unit which we call the autonomous nervous system. This system's counterpart we refer to as the endocrine system, and this I have written about in a number of my previous books. Everything should be in harmony, and if one little thing is not working efficiently, a problem will surely result.

The other day I realised once again that the body is like a human machine. I am a very poor driver and there are not many people who volunteer to be a passenger in my car. I mostly keep to back roads with very little traffic. My car is nineteen years old but has less than 40,000 miles on the clock. The other day, as I drove from home to the clinic, everything started to pack up. The battery light was on and the petrol indicator flashed. It looked as if every light on my dashboard had lit up, and I knew that something was badly wrong. How I made it to the clinic I don't know, but when I asked the gardener to have a look he was quick in telling me that the fanbelt had broken and I should consider myself lucky that I had even made it to the clinic. It made me think of this human machine and of how often stress has an influence on the whole machine when it threatens to come to a standstill. Not only will stress have an effect on the body mechanically, the effects are also felt mentally and emotionally. Consider the increase of cancer, degenerative diseases, ME, post-viral syndrome and so on.

People often ask if nowadays life is more difficult than previously, as stress is so widely experienced. Life has certainly become more complicated, and in earlier days, although people were also under stress, the pace of life was less demanding. The emotional trauma we experience today was probably not present.

It would be beneficial if we realised that the three bodies are involved when there is an attack on the counterpart of the autonomous nervous system which, as pointed out, is the endocrine system. This system consists of seven small glands which are extremely prone to stress. Consider the increase in cases of diabetes, pancreas problems, the many female hormonal complaints and malfunctioning of the thyroid gland. Other problems are even more stressful because the pineal gland does not excrete enough melatonin, especially as the pineal gland greatly affects the condition of ME patients. The adrenals are constantly under threat and the thymus gland is often incapable of coping, and therefore sometimes only partly functions. We must strive for harmony in this system and understand that life means movement, perfected in a rhythmic balance. Life means that we need a normal rhythm.

A few months ago, waking in the morning, I saw to my surprise that the entire landscape was covered with snow. During the night an unexpected snowstorm had covered the countryside with an unblemished white blanket. It was beautiful, and although it was not yet seven o'clock I woke my wife and suggested we go to the beach. We walked through beautiful snow-covered lanes to the beach, and looked towards the island of Arran, off the west coast of Scotland. The hills of Arran were entirely white, and they have never looked more beautiful. It was perfect harmony with creation. In the afternoon we went out again, but the beautiful snow-covered world of the morning had changed to a muddy scenery. Yet, when I looked over towards Arran, I noticed a beautiful rainbow that restored in my mind the harmony within nature.

There are seven endocrine glands, and the retina of the eye has seven light receptors. There are seven layers of light and there are seven basic steps in a musical octave. If these are out of balance, we have a problem. When we realise how easily harmony can be lost, it is necessary that our stress level is carefully watched. The nervous system controls all the functions of the body. If the motor system is disturbed, the sensory system is affected, and pain may result. The sympathetic nervous system is the superintendent of all bodily functions, and blood circulation is very important. A healthy circulation greatly depends on stress-free living, and a toxic condition, if allowed to take hold, can easily lead to degenerative disease.

My oldest patient, who lived to the age of a hundred and eight, was a typical example of healthy living. She experienced plenty of stress in her life; widowed before the age of fifty, she was left with thirteen children. She had very little money to live on and yet she brought up her children in an exemplary manner. When I first met her some thirty years ago, I concentrated on her circulatory system and told her that one is only as old as one's circulation. She took *Ginkgo biloba* (fifteen drops three times a day) and she knew how to cope with the stresses of life in a very sensible manner. It is important that we learn what stress can do to the body, and we should look for ways to relax in order to avoid the destructive effects of stress.

There are seven ways to reduce tension:

1. Take a physical break: Exercise, walk or otherwise interrupt your routine for five minutes or so at regular intervals throughout the working day.
2. Do not cheat on sleep: Try not to work at home, but if you must, stop at least an hour before you go to bed. Develop a hobby to take your mind off the job.
3. Learn to recognise stress: Watch for indicators like increased smoking, additional drinking and frequently disturbed sleep.
4. Stay with a problem: Do not switch to something else and leave it unsolved. Step back and reflect on it objectively before pursuing a conclusion.
5. Clarify your personal values: Recognise when it pays to fight and when it pays to yield.
6. Face up to your tensions: Accept the fact that you have them and work at ways to reduce them. This will help reduce organic effects.
7. Plan happy times with your family: Do things together that could provide you all with happy memories. Your husband or wife deserves the same consideration. Call home regularly when you're away on a trip, especially in the mornings.

This is a good start, and if you want to de-stress your life I can wholeheartedly recommend some breathing exercises, such as the Hara breathing method mentioned in a previous chapter. Have a good stretch, think positively, have plenty of sleep, take physical exercise, and enjoy yourself. At several times during the day, do some breathing exercises. This will help to cleanse as well as strengthen the body.

- Find a quiet place to sit down, with the back as straight as possible.
- Rest the left wrist on the right knee.
- Close the eyes and inhale normally.
- Close the right nostril with the right thumb, inhaling fully.
- Pause and exhale to the count of two.
- Block the left nostril using the little finger.
- Inhale and hold the breath to the count of ten.
- Release the thumb and exhale fully through the right nostril.
- Count to five.
- Keeping the left nostril closed, inhale through the right nostril to the count of two.
- Close both nostrils and count to eight.
- Release the left nostril, exhale and count to five.

A good selection of relaxation exercises can be found in my book *Body Energy*. Ensure that you follow a good stress-free diet, by which I mean avoid high-protein foods such as meat and eggs and make sure that carbohydrates are in balance. More advice can be found in my book *Nature's Gift of Food*.

Relaxation and breathing exercises, swimming, walking and cycling are all good for relaxation, and this will be helpful in coping with and overcoming stress. You might take JayVee tablets, and *Avena sativa* is also a recommended remedy. Start the day with a plate of porridge, which is a balanced food for a nervous constitution. Relax and roll with the tensions of life.

When people talk about tension, they usually think of mental tension, yet a muscle is capable of contraction and relaxation. In muscular spasms, the blood is squeezed out of the spastic muscle and oxygen cannot get to the tissue. Nature then gives its warning, which we experience as pain. It is an established fact that everything in nature is in a state of molecular tension, and that nothing stands still. Stillness is death and destruction.

Tension is a natural state of being. It is the most important factor in physical life, and it is responsible for the birth of form, controlling the harmonious distribution of energy through the body. It is this state of tension that preserves the integrity of form. Molecular construction of anything, be it animate or inanimate, is entirely dependent on this very natural law of tension. Call it life, health, energy or what you will, it is the factor which prevents molecules from flying into space. The tensile strength of a human cell is an electrical phenomenon and is allied to its frequency or rate of vibration. When this is altered by riotous living, the frequency and tension is altered. The end result is disease and disharmony.

Tension as we know it is muscular in nature, whether it be produced by cold weather, when we automatically tense ourselves, emotional stimuli or something else.

Tension, inner conflict, emotional upsets and so on are the causes of most functional disease, and these factors, when they persist, actually precipitate soluble calcium from the bloodstream into the joints. Call it by any name – it all ends in visceral motor tension. The results are arthritis, rheumatism, lumbago and other similar afflictions. This is called the negative miracle. On the other hand, the positive miracle is to supplant the latter with emotions such as joy and happiness, which are ideal conditions for survival.

Contraction of muscle is due to nervous impulses passing via a spinal nerve trunk to the nerve endings of the muscle. In a normal person this contraction is followed by relaxation, mainly due to exercise, which improves the metabolism and also increases the circulation of the blood flowing through the muscle, thus giving the muscle strength. When the nerves, through disease or injury, are no longer able to conduct these nerve impulses, in most cases muscle contraction becomes impossible. When a muscle remains contracted, the result is fatigue, pain and other harmful effects. Its supply of oxygen is cut off, and the blood and lymph are squeezed out of the affected tissue. What happens is that the muscle fibres contract violently but fail to relax properly, thus preventing blood and oxygen from reaching the muscle. This stressful state is considered by many doctors to end in muscle contraction or spasm. Factors like worry, fear and anxiety can bring on tension in muscles, and this leads to the names given to diseases such as fibrositis, neuritis and so on.

It is not generally known that asthma attacks are also due to a spasm which, when the lungs are about to evacuate the air inhaled, prevents expiration or breathing out by dilating the alveoli of the lungs and contracting the bronchial tubes. This complaint makes the life of the sufferer pure torment. Angina pectoris is essentially caused by a spasm which obstructs the coronary arteries, the arteries which convey food and oxygen to the cardiac muscles, so that the blood can no longer reach the tissue of the body.

It is worth noting that the sympathetic nervous system reaches all organs and controls blood circulation to all parts of the body. We should also remember that the nervous system controls all muscular effort, to which stimulation of the ganglion of impar and the perineum are the key.

Muscle spasm draws the tendons, ligaments and bones out of alignment. Just replacing or correcting a misaligned bone is merely a palliative move; these corrections never stay put for long. We should understand that muscles pull the bones or vertebrae out of place; bones do not suddenly get misaligned by themselves. No matter what the complaint, be it lumbago, a slipped disc, rheumatism, torticolis or female complaints, the release of muscles in a spasmodic state is of prime importance.

Without the relaxation of the primary, spastic set of muscles, no blood can flow to or from this locked area. The sympathetic reflexes govern the blood supply and must be first released through the ganglion of impar. Release of the spasm is always the primary requisite of any correction or relief of pain. The blood must be allowed to flow into this stagnant area and carry away the accumulated debris of solid acid crystals and their deposits in the cell structures before the muscles can contract without pain and spasm. Should any structural or spinal correction be attempted at this stage, the resulting pain and reaction will always be bad. This principle holds good for any forceful correction.

Anxiety neurosis changes the urine to alkaline. You can prove this for yourself by testing. When there is too much alkalinity, it paves the way for disease in the body. Bacteria of all strains flourish in an alkaline base, so all present-day tensions, frustrations, fears, phobias and repressions tend to create excessive alkalinity over a period of time. In other words, by negative thought you have changed the frequency of the wavelength of the normal cell structure within the organism. Added to this we have too much protein keeping the human body in continual high gear. Unfortunately, the rat race often demands this in these modern times.

Where does this lead us to? An easy and almost miraculous way to offset this is to stimulate the positive and negative ends of the sympathetic chain or ganglion. When a positive thought is carried long enough, it is propelled by the cosmic law of attraction to the negative or material plane and becomes a reality to the person who has formulated it. The triangle is complete. It is the same with the positive and negative ends of the sympathetic chain or ganglion. The positive and negative are stimulated and the break or fuse affecting the organism in question is repaired. Harmony exists once again, and thus the human triangle of balance is complete. The positive, negative and neutral are co-ordinated.

Chapter 13

ADDICTION ~ SELF-WILL

had a new patient who was a successful businessman with a beautiful and loyal wife, attractive and clever children, a magnificent home and a Rolls-Royce. He created the impression of being a successful and stable character, and yet, with the world at his feet, he could not control one thing, and that was drink. Addiction to alcohol was his problem, and although everybody was supportive, he could not overcome it. His mother-in-law had persuaded him to see me. She had spoken to me about his case and I asked her how, if no one else was able to get through to him, she could hope that I might succeed. She said that with my experience with people in similar circumstances I might be able to make him see common sense. We talked quite a bit, but I soon realised that I was not making any progress. We did, however, agree to meet again. The next meeting we arranged for an evening when I had no other appointments.

At this meeting we talked as friends, not as patient and practitioner. He spoke about his life and he gradually started to trust me. He spoke about the happiness in his home life and I found it hard to pinpoint the foundation of his problem until I asked him some questions about his youth. He told me that he had had a very strict religious upbringing and that he greatly admired his parents, who were always ready to lend a hand to other people. He had tried to follow in their footsteps, but when he was about ten or eleven years old something had happened that changed his life forever. As his parents were very supportive of their church, they had invited one of the missionaries who was on a home-visit from abroad to stay with them. He used their house as a base while he travelled around and gave talks about his work.

My patient's parents then went away for a weekend, leaving their son in the charge of the missionary. They got on well together and had long chats. As usual, the missionary spoke with the boy about his experiences abroad, a subject which greatly fascinated the youngster as he was at a very impressionable age. They talked about religion and, once the missionary had gained the boy's confidence, the conversation strayed on to sex. The boy was very naïve, probably because of a strict upbringing, and had no idea of what was happening. The missionary went with him to his bedroom and spoke to him about the facts of life, quoting sections from the Bible intimating that there was no harm in a growing physical intimacy. The boy, without realising what was happening, consented, but it was not until the next day that shame set in. The missionary, however, impressed upon him that he was never to speak of what had taken place, because he would bring major problems upon himself and his family.

The boy carried this guilty secret, and gradually the realisation of what he had been drawn into dawned upon him. Eventually he broached the subject with his parents, who out of misplaced shame and protectiveness towards their religion instructed him to forget it had ever happened and never to mention it to anyone. Due to the secrecy, he suppressed the events in his mind, but the realisation of what had happened was too much for him to cope with. Moreover, just before he was due to be married he was nearly embroiled in a similar situation, although he was able to turn his back on it. The security of his love for his fiancée and her love for him gave him the strength to turn his back on the past. However, one day he again met the missionary, and his reaction was so fierce that it placed his nervous system under severe pressure. The old memories and shame were raked up – and that was when he turned to drink.

This information was slowly drawn out of my patient, who hesitantly answered my questions. Nevertheless, because of the kind of person he was, he opened himself up to such an extent that it was clear that this unfortunate experience in his youth was the underlying reason for his drink problem. He had never been able to talk about it and therefore no one had been able to exonerate him from any blame. It had caused an imbalance in his life that made him turn to drink, especially if there was any stress in his life. He candidly told me that in moments of peace, or when he was on holiday, he did not drink.

This story was revealing, and it made me think of the many addicts I meet in the course of my work. I think not only of people addicted to drink, but also those addicted to cigarettes, drugs and over-eating. Many times I meet people who at the peak of their life become over-anxious and start to drink, either to gain courage or to give them some extra confidence. With misgivings I remember a young man who sought my help. I failed to help him, because he had convinced himself that he was in control of his need for alcohol. I knew better, and I told him that because his liver was already affected, it would be too late unless he took drastic steps very quickly. Unfortunately this man died young, all because of his indulgence and his refusal to recognise what was an alcohol addiction.

This brings me to a young woman who told me that twenty years ago, when she was in her mid-teens, she experienced involuntary movements of her limbs, as if she was not in control of her body movements. It was all the more frightening because this happened when she was fully awake. A psychiatrist explained that half her brain was asleep and half was awake, but she instinctively knew that there must be more to it than that. Then she experienced a terrible sensation of something trying to get into her body. It started with a dreadful noise in her head. She clenched her teeth and was shaking physically, imagining that her mind had left her body and that she was a mere presence in the room, an onlooker. When she tried to tell her parents of this weird experience, she was ridiculed. I can well imagine that she struggled trying to describe such a sensation, but the refusal of her parents to listen to her did nothing to reassure her. In her panic she sought a way to dull the strength of her emotions, and she found that drink helped her to dull the memory of these sensations. She went to an alternative therapist who advised that in order to overcome her drink problem she needed distraction. Actually, he got her interested in reflexology, and in time she developed a great skill in this therapy. Once she had gained confidence she became a great help to others. She poured all her energy into developing her skills and she became a very successful therapist.

For a long time she had been able to resist alcohol, but in a weak moment at a party she again took a drink, and this was the beginning of a major lapse into alcoholism. This proves the truth of the saying 'Once an alcoholic, always an alcoholic'. One cannot afford to give into drink if this has once been diagnosed as a problem. Acupuncture treatment often helps to overcome problems relating to alcoholism. For many people, membership of a self-help group such as Alcoholics Anonymous is invaluable, but not everyone is prepared or able to participate in therapy at a group level. These people quite often seek the help of a therapist on an individual basis, and these tend to be the people who visit me at my clinics. Generally, for the treatment of an alcohol dependency I concentrate on nutritional supplements such as zinc, vitamin E, Ginsavita and vitamin C for detoxification. With these remedies, together with guidance and support, I am able to help most of my patients with their addiction. There is certainly much that can be done. Finding the root of the problem and then using the correct remedies and techniques can help an alcoholic overcome his or her addiction.

You are what you eat and what you drink, and a will within yourself is much stronger than you can believe. I see this often with smokers. Nicotine can actually be much more addictive than alcohol, and not only is it equally destructive in the human body, it is also the cause of a form of self-poisoning. The physical system is under attack because of the waste material of nicotine, so that it can adversely affect one's health very severely, developing into serious and degenerative disease. If people understood how little nicotine is needed to poison the system, they would surely think twice about smoking. Yet it is often insecurity in younger years that makes them reach out for a prop that becomes a curse, and before they know it they are hooked.

Again, much can be done to overcome nicotine addiction. Smoking is a foul and unhealthy habit, and I am pleased to see that nowadays it is also considered an extremely anti-social pastime. It is certainly a habit that sooner or later will takes its toll.

With acupuncture, not only can the habit be broken, but the desire to smoke can also be controlled. This does not, of course, mean that will-power or self-control is not required. If the smoker could only see what a pathologist sees every day of his working life, it would be a good lesson about the damage to health that is caused by this habit.

Although acupuncture treatment may be helpful in breaking the habit, a single cigarette may sometimes be enough for a smoker to revert to his old habits, just as one drink is often enough for a reformed alcoholic.

As part of the therapy to help people to stop smoking, it is important for the smoker to realise the benefits of stopping: better health, chest, lungs, taste, smell and skin, and a lot more money in the pocket. If this is kept in mind, it may help to strengthen the smoker in his or her determination not to smoke again. I often prescribe the homoeopathic remedy Tabacum as a substitute for nicotine. Sometimes peppermint or chewing gum also helps to break the habit. Many of my patients who have stopped smoking admit that they feel much happier when they have been able to break this addiction. They are also healthier, and are likely to live longer with a better quality of life. I always remind smokers that people aren't born with chimneys on their heads.

This brings me to the many people I have treated with sugar addictions. Because there is no social stigma attached, this is often an even more difficult addiction than the others. Weak people will whisper to themselves that this one little bit of cake can do them no harm, or that this one biscuit or ice-cream is no problem, because they will do without tomorrow. Huge sums of money are spent on weight reduction. The slimming classes in our clinics are very successful, because here too we apply acupuncture treatment to break the habit and the craving. Again, however, the motivation must come from the patient. If patients are vain enough to want to be slim, they must be willing to make sacrifices. But even then help and support may be needed, and my book *Realistic Weight Control* is full of advice to help people to change their eating habits.

I once had a female patient who admitted that she was addicted to a particular brand of chocolate. She actually did very well and lost several stone in weight, for which she was praised by her family. They were very supportive and appreciated her courage and will-power. Then she encountered a domestic problem which caused her a lot of stress. Unaware of her problem, someone presented her with a box of chocolates in a gesture of kindness. Realising the temptation this represented, she immediately threw them into the bin. When her husband had not come home at bedtime, however, she had no one to share her concerns with, and she became so uptight that the word 'chocolate' kept going through her mind. She could not think of anything else. Although she had locked the windows and doors of the house for the night, she could not get the thought out of her mind that in the bin outside there was this tempting box of chocolates. She got out of bed, made her way downstairs and unlocked the back door. In the dark she groped around in the bin until she found the box, took it into the house and ate the entire contents.

Contrary to what people may say, the problems of excess body weight are rarely caused by health problems. They are much more likely to be caused by eating more food than is needed by the body, often combined with insufficient physical exercise. The external factors are affluence, persuasion of advertising, pace of life, giving up smoking, marriage problems and general confusion and lack of confidence. Internal factors are lack of will-power, self-control and patience, boredom, loneliness, fear, worry, anxiety, eating for comfort, self-indulgence, wrong mental attitude to food, insecurity, temptations and compulsions.

Drug addiction is different. Rarely does the drug addict realise what is involved. A drug's influence makes us feel important, daring, adventurous and capable of anything. When I think of the many ruined lives I have seen and the struggle that the addict goes through to reach the freedom of living without drugs, I feel so terribly sorry for those who are completely and utterly addicted. Usually it starts with soft drugs, in the full belief that they are non-addictive, but too often this can be the beginning of the end. Don't let anyone tell you otherwise, because it is a popular myth that soft drugs are not addictive and will not lead on to hard drugs.

Positive help is necessary, and I am grateful every time I can help an addict to overcome his or her addiction, preventing many more lives from being ruined. The sad reality is that drug addiction not only ruins the life of the addict but also affects the lives of the parents, partners and offspring. There would not be enough room in this book to tell you of the many traumas I have witnessed, mostly with young people, in my efforts to help them try to kick the habit. Life becomes very desperate, as our permissive society encourages indulgence.

Drug addiction led a young patient of mine, who was a successful businessman, near to bankruptcy. He recognised that he had reached a critical point, and with his remaining will-power and all the help I could give him we battled to overturn his addiction. So near to total failure, he fully co-operated, and with acupuncture treatments and homoeopathic and herbal remedies I managed to help him. I still see him occasionally and it does me good to know that he is happy in his life and work.

Nevertheless, I am shocked about the general attitude to drug abuse. A lawyer phoned me not so long ago and told me that he would pay a great deal of money for a report about a young man who had mugged an old lady in an Underground station. He stole her bag to provide him with money to buy drugs. The parents of this young man told the lawyer that they would pay what was required to keep him out of prison. The lawyer asked me if I was prepared to make a statement saying that I would treat him, in order to keep him out of prison. Of course I was willing to take him on as a patient, but I could not promise to be successful because I cannot give anyone the will-power that is required to beat such an addiction. I would do my best to help him, but without his commitment I would be certain to fail.

An addictive nature can lead to the destruction of oneself and others. It is not easy if there is no will-power, and positive thinking is necessary. Prayer and meditation are good exercises to develop self-will. Breathing exercises are helpful too, and taking responsibility for life should be uppermost in the mind. Thomas Edison failed nine thousand nine hundred and ninety-nine times to create a light bulb. Someone once asked him if he could bear to fail the ten thousandth time, and he looked at him with disbelief. He exclaimed that ten thousand failures had taught him nine thousand nine hundred and ninety-nine ways of how to create the perfect light bulb. In fact, he did succeed the ten thousandth time, and without the many failures he would not have been successful. Positive actions with exercise or meditation will result in success.

A short while ago I again saw a person whom I had been trying to help when he had come to me with a glue-sniffing addiction. I told him that if he did some exercises that are helpful in strengthening one's will-power, he could overcome his addiction. He had managed and was quite excited that he had succeeded. He was also grateful that he now felt so much better in himself, not just because he had overcome his addiction to glue, but also because he had grown as a person, realising that it was largely due to his self-control.

It is so important that an addict recognises the need for help. Will-power needs to be exercised, and this can be encouraged with positive actions. Utilising this will-power makes us feel much stronger, and especially when we manage to overcome struggles from the past, the victory proves that these addictions can be over-come. Patients tell me how much better they feel and not only physically. Mentally they have grown into stronger characters, having faced the pitfalls of life and overcome them.

Chapter 14

●

FRUSTRATION ∼ FULFILMENT

A patient across the desk told me she was so frustrated because she could not get on with the job she was doing. I felt truly sorry for her, because she came across as a determined lady but I could see that she was frustrated by obstacles that stopped her reaching her goal. She was a middle-aged lady, very capable, and her work was important to her. She wanted to get on and make something of her life, and she gave the impression that she craved fulfilment. This was currently beyond her reach, because the job that was entrusted to her restricted her initiative and did not give her the chance of self-development. This attitude from the management had made her ill, and she was nervous and uptight.

First of all she needed to learn to relax. When I mentioned relaxation exercises, I got the quick answer that she had done all that and that nothing had helped. Her entire reaction was negative, and she explained that she had tried everything possible to counter her frustrations but that it was not in her power to effect the changes that were required. I countered by telling her that frustrations can last for a while but will not last forever, either because something would happen that would change the circumstances and remove the ground for her frustrations or because she would find something else to replace the work that frustrated her so badly at the moment. A chance to change her job presented itself, and, indeed, she became a much happier and more contented person. She shed the frustrations that had blocked her progress in her previous job and she reached a much higher level of fulfilment.

This made me think of a letter from a slightly younger person, a patient whom I had grown to like very much because it was obvious that she really wanted to work at overcoming her frustrations and, moreover, she wanted to put back into her life what she thought she owed it. She wrote me a long letter in which she said that she felt that my book *Body Energy* raised a concept which she claimed not to understand, but that it helped her to accept an experience she had had when she was nineteen years old, which she wanted to share with me. She had just started her first job, working in a bank, and she was sent on a training course in Edinburgh. At the end of the day she returned to the railway station but was concerned about meeting the bus in Glasgow to take her home. She decided to find a seat in the front carriage of the train and run for the bus as soon as the train pulled into the station in Glasgow. As she walked on to the platform, she suddenly experienced the most intense pain in her feet. She decided to get on the train and when she felt better she would work her way through the carriages to the front, hoping that the floor of the carriages would cushion the impact on her painful feet better than the concrete of the platform. Clearly intending to walk the entire length of the train, she came to a point when she entered the second carriage from the front. She took a few steps forward and stopped, turned round and made her way back to the carriage she had just left. She wrote that she had no reason; it was more of an intuitive than a conscious decision. She felt drawn towards a specific seat that had been vandalised and had its stuffing spilling out everywhere.

As she sat down she wondered what had come over her, because the train was practically empty, and, still thinking of her connecting bus, she decided to get up and make her way to the front, as she had intended to do in the first place. She never made it to the front carriage, because as the train approached one of the stations where it was due to stop, the brakes were applied, a screeching sound filled the railway carriage and, struck with horror, she realised the train was out of control. When it started to tilt, she was petrified and wondered if this was the way she was going to die. She wrote that her life flashed before her, and thoughts of her family and grandparents whirled in her mind. She remembered that her parents were away on a well-deserved holiday, and that if anything happened to her it would ruin their first holiday together since their family had grown up. She was thinking of her boyfriend and their plans for the future when something pierced the window on the other side of the aisle. Although she at first thought it was a tree, she soon realised that it was a train carriage, presumably because the train had jack-knifed. As she was showered with glass, she refused to believe that she was going to be killed and willed the destruction to stop . . . and the intruding train carriage stopped inches from her.

The carriage had come three or four feet into her carriage, the table had collapsed and dusty air swirled around. Outside, bodies were strewn everywhere, having been thrown from the two carriages in front that had completely derailed. With great effort, crawling on hands and knees, she made her way up the embankment, where she saw bodies and debris scattered everywhere. Although she wanted to help, she was in no fit state, and she just sat at the top of the embankment, thanking God for her miraculous escape. She had intended to make her way to the front of the train, but she felt that God had somehow stopped her from getting there. Travellers who were not injured or only slightly wounded helped those who were worse, and these signs of humanity, selflessness and compassion made her grateful for being alive. At the same time she wondered sadly why it required an accident to bring out these compassionate traits in people. Later it became clear that most of the passengers in the first carriage had been killed and those in the second carriage had suffered severe injuries and were hospitalised, some for a very long time.

In her letter, the girl continued that she had tried to rationalise these events, but with little success, and therefore she concluded that her guardian angel must

have been looking after her. She wondered if her experience meant anything to me in my reflection of energy.
Whenever she thinks of this experience, she realises that
if she had not followed this strange intuition and turned
back from the second carriage when she did, she might
also have been a fatality in this train derailment. She is
determined to pay more attention to her intuition in
future. In her private life she had at that time suffered a
lot of frustration, and she wondered if this experience
had to take place to make her aware of the futility of her
frustrations.

Sometimes it needs such experiences to find fulfilment. Life is full of frustrations. We meet them daily. We
are, for instance, frustrated with a job that is not carried
out according to instructions. Most of us will have
experienced that when we have been let down by
tradesmen, either when they do not turn up when they
are supposed to or when we are not satisfied with the
quality of their work. I suffer unduly from frustrations
when I want to see a patient improve and it is taking
longer than expected. Dr Vogel often told me that I had
to learn to be more patient than the patient, but this is
not in my character. It frustrates me to know that
although I want to see a patient get better it can be so
slow. With regard to frustration, however, the winners
are those who are patient and who accept that by frustrating themselves they cannot change the situation.

Because I have travelled extensively, I have learnt the
frustrations of delayed flights, late trains, motorway
congestion and pile-ups, and delay due to poor weather
conditions. I hate being late for appointments, and I
equally dislike being kept waiting by someone else who

is late for an appointment, irrespective of the reason. Something I realised myself in life was that I had to learn to cope with frustrations. We cannot hurry a plane, neither can we stop a train. Life will follow its own route and go at its own pace, and we must learn to cope with it, however difficult it may be. We just have to accept life, including the frustrations it brings us.

On a wintry day a frustrated father came to me with his beautiful daughter. I had known the family for years and I could see he was a very troubled man. His face showed how worried he was. He told me that his daughter had a great future but that suddenly her life had come to a standstill because of a condition that was diagnosed as lateral sclerosis, an incurable disease. When I heard the story I feared that there was no hope for this beautiful girl who was in the bloom of her life. I concluded that in the short time she had left, life would not be kind to her. She seemed to accept it as fate, however, and I have always envied her tremendous faith in accepting a situation not of her own making. I advised her to the best of my ability and moved heaven and earth to help her, and the best doctors and specialists were also called in. I visited her at home at a time when she was completely unable to move any of her limbs, her speech deteriorating rapidly. I came home very upset.

The next day her sister came to see me. This is when the hurt penetrated even more deeply, because as I spoke to her sister I sensed that she was also suffering from the same wasting disease. She too was a very attractive girl and delighted because she was expecting her first baby. With hope in his eyes, her husband pleaded with me to help her. I accompanied them to a specialist to find out if there was anything that could be done. We soon had confirmation that she had the same mysterious illness with which her sister had been diagnosed. There was yet another victim. My frustration was beyond bounds. I had to help these girls, but it was all to no avail. With God's help we managed to sustain her so that she could be delivered of her baby, and every time I see this young child I feel grateful that I was able to help the mother. The few months she had with her baby she was so happy. She died because she chose not to have the operation that her sister had opted for, which kept her alive, albeit artificially. The married sister reached complete fulfilment through the birth of her baby. She overcame her frustrations thanks to her great faith, and she died peacefully. Her sister, however, is still alive, and whenever I see her I am aware of a fulfilment in her life, indicating that she is at peace with her condition. Her great faith in God has never been shaken.

Tragically, I discovered that the probable cause was heavy metal poisoning. When these girls were young they used to play in a sand-pit in their back garden. Unknown to their parents, a neighbour who was experimenting with heavy chemicals had a dump just the other side of the fence. Polluted soil is thought to have drained into the sand-pit, causing damage to the nerve tissues of these children. Severe attacks on the nervous systems of these young children during their formative years were to take their toll.

Frustrations come and go. While attending to these two girls during their illnesses, I admired the way they coped with the cruel blow life had dealt them. In the knowledge that they would not be getting better, and knowing that the end was near, they accepted their fate. Possibly the worst frustrations were experienced by the parents, who had to stand by and support their children to the very end. They had good reason to be enormously proud of them, and this justifiable pride brought fulfilment in its own way.

Fulfilment in work and in life is tremendously important, and it should be recognised that most disturbances are of our own making. Any disruption in life disturbs the harmony between our Creator and ourselves.

Chapter 15

SENILITY ~ COMPASSION

My parents were compassionate and always ready to help others. They had a sensible approach to health all through their lives. However, when my mother was eighty-five years old the first signs of senility became recognisable. I was worried, because she had always prayed to God to grant her soundness of mind, as she called it. When she began to deteriorate she became a little lazy, and sometimes found it hard to make the effort to come up with the right answer. My wife often worked with her, and her patience and insistence helped. But as my mother grew older still, senility became unavoidable. Although she still had her clear moments, it upset me to hear her confusing facts with fiction. She still told us stories, but more and more often they were confused and irrelevant.

A number of friends with sharp and clear intellects reached a stage in their lives when senility took over. I have often wondered why a sound mind deteriorates to such an extent. The mind is a wonderful thing, but it is also very complex, and in old age the arteries start to deteriorate and the mind may become confused. It is difficult to know how to prevent this from happening. A healthy diet containing the ninety-one essential nutrients may help, and if there are known deficiencies, nutritional supplements may be beneficial. Raw foods contain many valuable enzymes. Researchers have concluded that the American diet contains twenty times too much sodium because of table salt. Other adverse influences are food additives such as colourings and preservatives; packaging labels should be studied, especially when deterioration of the mind sets in. Being healthy includes ridding the body of contamination, toxicity and other pollutants that interfere with the system.

Oral chelation therapy such as FLW contains the nutrients necessary for a sound mind and is often helpful when the first signs of senility become apparent. Chelation therapy can be safely administered. It was first introduced in 1948 in the United States, containing several vitamins, minerals and trace elements, to combat the effects of lead poisoning. However, in trials it was discovered that it also lowered the cholesterol level, and it is even thought to emulsify or dissolve loose particles present in the arteries. Much research has been undertaken to substantiate or refute such claims, but unfortunately the controversy surrounding the benefits of such therapy still continues. For me, however, the proof can be found in the enthusiastic testimonies of patients who have used this therapy – and their testimonies are virtually unanimous in their praise. Results cannot be disputed.

Chelation therapy is actually a nutritional remedy and an effective combination of chelating nutrients obtained from natural sources. It can be administered by injection, but oral chelation is also available. No adverse side-effects have been reported and it appears that chelation therapy can effect a reversal of the hardening of the arteries, instead strengthening the bones and the teeth.

Obviously, chelation therapy has attracted a great deal of interest. In recent years it also captured the attention of the well-known health practitioner and Nobel prize winner Dr Linus Pauling, the great advocate of vitamin C, who endorsed chelation therapy by saying, 'I think it is an invaluable treatment for many patients as an alternative to therapy, not just for the heart by-pass patient, but for patients with a variety of problems.' I have noticed that it has become widely accepted that chelation therapy reduces toxic metal deposits, high blood pressure, cholesterol, calcium deposits and, sometimes, kidney stones, and that it greatly improves the circulation, skin texture, liver function, hearing, vision and general well-being. So, all in all, it has given tremendous hope to people with many different problems.

It is, of course, up to the individual when and how to take action, as ultimately we are all responsible for our own health. There is no single 'miracle' ingredient available that will do the trick unsupported. Rather, it is the synergistic total of all ingredients working together and supporting each other that is vital. In my experience, the daily intake of each supplementary nutrient necessary to produce the vascular cleansing response is most effectively combined in the FLW formula, which is made up as follows:

Vitamin A (palmitate)	3,333iu
Vitamin D3	67iu
Vitamin E (d-alpha tocopheryl succ.)	60iu
Vitamin C (ascorbic acid)	500mg
Vitamin B (thiamine hydrochloride)	18mg
Vitamin B2 (riboflavin)	3mg
Vitamin B6 (pyridoxine hydrochloride)	15mg
Vitamin B12 (cobalamin)	16mcg
Niacin	7mg
Niacinamide	2mg
Pantothenic Acid (d-calcium pantothenate)	33mg
Folic Acid	0.06mg
Biotin	5mcg
Choline (bitartrate)	66mg
Inositol	4mg
DL-Methionine	16mg
Calcium (carbonate)	42mg
Magnesium (oxide)	42mg
Potassium (chloride)	42mg
Iron (ferrous fumarate)	1.34mg
Iodine (potassium iodide)	0.03mg
Manganese (gluconate)	0.8mg
Zinc (gluconate)	2.5mg
Chromium (proteinate)	13mcg
Selenium (proteinate)	20mcg

Non-medical ingredients

PABA	10mg
Betaine Hydrochloride	13mg
Lemon Bioflavonoids	10mg
L-Cysteine Hydrochloride	66mg
Thymus Concentrate	6mg
Spleen Concentrate	6mg
Adrenal Concentrate	4mg

This is indeed an impressive formula and one that can be taken with other medication without adverse effects. The results will not be noticeable overnight, but gradually one will become aware of an improvement. This remarkable formula has also proved to be of great help in the treatment of other problems such as headaches, intestinal gas, nausea and diarrhoea. Moreover, no toxicity has been shown from its use. Knowing that our drinking water has not been up to standard for quite some time because of chemical additives and pollution in general, I therefore sometimes recommend the FLW chelation formula in cases where I suspect excess toxicity.

More information and evidence on chelation therapy can be found in my book *Heart and Blood Circulation Problems*.

Ginkgo biloba, a wonderful herbal remedy, is known to keep the mind fresh and stimulated. I remember working with Dr Vogel in the Far East when an elderly Korean man picked a ginkgo leaf and started chewing it. No one could tell us how old he was but he was thought to be over a hundred years old, and he claimed that the ginkgo leaf had kept his mind alert. It is encouraging to see that the leaf has the form of a brain, and this heavy leaf is held by a little stem which reminds me of the stem of the brain. The shape of the leaf could be considered a message from nature that it is beneficial for the brain. In many cases of senility this wonderful herb, in combination with FLW, has been of great benefit.

When concentration becomes difficult, Cerebrum, which is mineral therapy in a homoeopathic solution, may be beneficial. Concentration Essence, a flower essence containing a wide variety of herbs and flowers, also provides support for the concentration. The first signs of senility are recognised when the patient forgets names and incidents, and immediate action should be taken to stimulate the brain. We kept trying to motivate my mother when she lost her memory and sharpness of mind, and every time we encouraged and motivated her we could see that her brain worked a little better, because we challenged it.

Compassion is necessary when dealing with senility. A while ago I had a lady in my consulting-room and it was clear that her family was running out of patience. The hope in her eyes was very touching. When I questioned her about her lifestyle, her answers initially made good sense, but after a little while her answers became confused. I can imagine that it is hard for someone who has to care for a senile person not to lose patience, and in the eyes of this patient I could see that she was pleading for reassurance and compassion. It sounds easier than it is in reality to be compassionate when coping with a senile person, as it is very demanding, yet we must never forget that this state of mind is not of the person's own choosing. The causes of senility may be numerous and not necessarily related to the stresses of life, yet it is very necessary that in such instances the patient feels that he or she is having the care and interest that any human being deserves.

I have often noticed that senile patients receive comfort from something as simple as having their hand held. The human hand is trained from infancy to express the thoughts or purpose of the mind which controls it. The hand is the tool on which the mind depends when it wants to do anything practical. Thoughts of action naturally turn to the hand for their expression. Babies use their hands long before they learn to walk. The savage who has only a few words in his vocabulary depends on hands to express his thoughts. The hand ministers and carries aid. The hand lifts the fallen, ministers to the sick and is peculiarly the organ of expression for the good wishes of the kindly disposed. When we are hurt we instinctively place a hand upon the injured part. When another suffers and we sympathise, we instinctively use the hand to soothe pain. Clasped hands are the universal pledge of friendship and goodwill. From the earliest dawn of civilisation, the hand has been used in the most sacred ceremonies. The hand is the natural organ of expression and its actions are mental symbols to which man has learned to respond through untold ages of experience and adaptation.

Holding someone's hand is a great comfort and emotional support, as senile patients can be lost within themselves. It shows compassion. We have to learn that, although their minds may appear absent, senile people still need our help, and they still deserve our love and compassion.

Chapter 16

WORK RESENTMENT ~ JOB SATISFACTION

I feel extremely sorry for people who suffer from resentment at work. They are usually cynical and unhappy in their private lives, and work becomes a millstone around their necks. It is easy to say that this is the time to forget it and leave it, but not everyone gets the opportunity to move on to something else.

When I was involved in medical trials on arthritis and rheumatism treatment therapies, we had sixty patients undergoing orthodox treatment while sixty patients were treated with alternative methods. The orthodox approach was to concentrate on allergies, infections or inherited factors, prescribing standard treatment according to orthodox methods. Not one of the rheumatologists I worked with considered the relationship between the three bodies of man, yet emotional stress such as jealousy, unhappiness in marriage or work resentment can have a major bearing on health. During these trials I discovered to my great astonishment how many people suffered from emotional stress such as work resentment and how many people could not respond to change. Nowadays psychologists do their best to counsel those who suffer from work resentment and guide those who are unhappy in their work.

We must realise that the majority of our waking hours are spent at work, and if we are unhappy it is bound to affect our health. I remember a patient who was a garage foreman and very happy in his work until, because of his arthritis, he had to take a step down. He had a new supervisor and there was resentment between them. The result was that his arthritic condition deteriorated, because he resented going to work, and he became badly crippled. When I was able to help him leave this environment and become involved in some other work, his condition improved rapidly again. This man needed the mental stimulation of work, and his pride in his work gave him enjoyment and fulfilment. The difference was startling in his new job because he was happy in what he was doing. He got on with his new responsibilities, and his health flourished.

It makes me think of a practice where I once worked. It was a general practice and of the six doctors who worked there I was the eldest. I had joined the practice to provide alternative therapies. The senior partner of the practice was concerned about the mental attitude of a new doctor who had recently started. She was, indeed, the most unhappy person I had ever come across, and it was ascribed to work resentment. Because I was a bit older than the others, the senior practitioner asked me to talk to her to find out what was wrong. One day I plucked up the courage when I saw her sitting in her consulting-room, and I asked her how she was. In no uncertain terms she responded that it was none of my business. She obviously resented me as well as her work. I was not to be put off that easily, however, and I asked her why she was so unhappy. Again she replied that it was none of my business. Then I remarked that she gave the impression that she was unhappy at work, and she retorted that I would not be happy either if I was called out on house calls numerous times each day, many of them at night, for little or no reason. I wondered aloud why she had chosen this profession, because being a general practitioner is more of a calling than a job. Doctors have to get used to the fact that house calls are part of the job, as are interrupted nights. I am only too aware how frustrating it can be, but nevertheless it should not cause work resentment. If that is the case, the person is in the wrong profession.

She mellowed a little when I spoke to her about my own experiences, but nevertheless she felt that this was not the job for her. I told her that if she had reached that conclusion it would be better if she found something else to do, because if she did not see her work as a calling and a duty to help human suffering, she could not function well in this profession. I remarked on the positive aspect of her work and the job satisfaction she could experience when looking at it from a different perspective.

A few weeks later two of the doctors in the practice asked me what I had said to her, because she definitely appeared happier and more approachable. She smiled every now and then, and I assume that she had decided to tackle her job wholeheartedly once she had considered the options of giving up or getting on with it. This is often the case, because job satisfaction can only be ours if we give one hundred per cent of ourselves. Too often I see examples of people suffering the daily regime in order to receive their pay at the end of the week. Work then becomes a means of survival, as people's minds are not on their work and they have no job satisfaction. Work becomes a drudgery, and their working lives are spent in misery.

As a child I had a great interest in trains, and I spent a lot of time with one of my father's friends who was an engine-driver. This man took great pride in his locomotives, always making sure that the brass was shining and lovingly caring for his engine. It was the pride in his work that made him the man he was, and when he retired he did so with well-deserved honour.

Successful people are people with job satisfaction. I am all in favour of the work of discussion groups and psychologists who study unhappiness at work. So many people fall into a pattern of leaving work as early as possible, going for a drink or sitting in front of the television. To my way of thinking, this hardly constitutes a happy and healthy life. I cannot pretend to be a typical example, but although I am in my early sixties, a ninety-hour working week is a pleasure to me. I am proud and happy that I am still able to work, and the satisfaction of helping people who are in need is for me the greatest challenge possible. It is that which makes my job so special, and I am lucky, as job satisfaction is probably one of the greatest factors for good health.

In my lectures I always set aside time to answer questions from the public. One question was from a person who explained that he had no respect for his boss, as he considered him dishonest. The questioner wanted to know how he was expected to work for this person. I agreed that under those conditions it was difficult to perform well but, in fairness, you do not work to satisfy someone else; the work you do should be to satisfy your own standards. Confronting a boss like that may cause considerable problems, but if the man applied himself it would be recognised, and he might be offered another job that would be more rewarding.

When I was in Indiana in the United States, I stayed on a farm. During the night the weather was very windy and I was told a story about a farming couple who were looking for a reliable farm labourer. They interviewed several men and one of the applicants had little to say for himself except that he would do his best and that he was able to sleep on windy nights. They liked the look of him, and because he was strong and healthy they offered him the job. On a very stormy night, the husband and wife were concerned about possible damage to their property. That night they inspected the outbuildings and found that all windows and doors were securely locked and bolted in readiness for the storm. They found the farmhand fast asleep, and when they told him of their concern because of the bad weather he asked if they had found everything in order. After they had reassured him, he reminded them that when he was interviewed he had said that he could sleep in all weather conditions. In the knowledge that he had secured the buildings, he was able to sleep contentedly. It is satisfying to see people live up to their responsibilities in life. No matter how insignificant one's duty may appear, if it is done with pride it will result in job satisfaction. I am a great believer that if a job is worth doing, it is worth doing well.

Chapter 17

☯

MID-LIFE CRISIS ∼ HORMONAL BALANCE

M ost of you will agree that the mid-life crisis, for men as well as women, can cause great turmoil. It is a pity that at this stage in life many people seem to lose their direction, when this time of life can have such great attraction. Many men and women are happy to reach this stage, often having raised a family and been successful in their chosen career, and the richer for having experienced life. Unfortunately, only too often middle-aged men regret the loss of their youth, and decide on a last fling before it is too late. It is at this stage of life that many marriages fall apart. Too often this uncertainty in men coincides with a lack of direction in the lives of women, who see their children leaving home and feel as if they have lost their purpose in life. I find it very sad when I come across such situations. I have seen couples who have had a stable relationship for many years throw it all away because one partner experiences a mid-life crisis. I have seen and still see too many people in my clinics who are bereft at the loss of their partner during this stage of their lives, and in many this manifests itself as problems with health.

When I lecture, in America in particular, I am often asked how I feel about HRT, or Hormone Replacement Therapy. This preparation allegedly keeps us looking young, without wrinkles, and also re-energises us. It is a fact that for people over the age of fifty the sex drive is no longer as strong. However, it is also thought that at middle age one is no longer attractive to the opposite sex. This I regard as the greatest nonsense, as life then becomes more interesting. In all fairness, many men will agree that a mature woman is certainly much more appealing to a man. She may no longer have the fresh-ness of youth, but she has gained in character because she has experienced life. The same applies to men. Many young women prefer more mature men, because they represent stability and are more experienced than younger men who are still set on proving themselves.

Women are sometimes hesitant or reluctant to talk about their feelings, their fears and inhibitions, and the effects of a mid-life crisis or the menopause. Thankfully there is more openness today than in the days of our grandparents. Certainly, our grandmothers would rather have bitten off their tongues than admit to any-thing that could remotely be considered as a mid-life crisis or the menopause. In *Anthony and Cleopatra*, Shakespeare wrote that 'Age cannot wither her nor custom steal her infinite variety'.

The use of HRT started in New York in the '60s. Very

little was known of its side-effects, and although it claimed to have none, I have witnessed to my sorrow many cases of phlebitis, thrombosis and breast cancer where I feared the influence of HRT. Although I have sometimes prescribed HRT myself, it is only with reluctance, because there are so many alternative approaches to these problems available. Optivite and Gynovite Plus made by Nature's Best immediately spring to mind. A natural alternative HRT remedy is Phytogen from Enzymatic Therapy. This product has many properties to combat symptoms of the menopause and helps women to overcome problems that are quite common at this stage of life.

A great friend of mine in the United States, Dr Lynn Walker, wrote in one of her books, 'What is the prime of life? May it not be defined as a period of about twenty years in a woman's and thirty years in the life of a man?' This remark leads us to wonder why or how mid-life crises occur. In the Western world, when hormonal changes become apparent they are considered part of the ageing process in the lives of men and women, and a healthy diet is thought to be very important. For that reason I have written about the dietary requirements for such conditions in my book *Menopause*. In Chinese medicine the menopause is explained and treated as a blood deficiency problem, and balance is often regained with the aid of acupuncture treatment or with cranial osteopathy.

Much can be done to maintain or regain the hormonal balance that allows women to go through the menopause quickly and naturally. One of the most common symptoms is hot flushes, and these are reportedly experienced by two-thirds of Western women. Salvia, or Menosan, is a fresh herbal extract and an excellent remedy for hot flushes. Equally, I have seen some very good results when patients took MNP Formula. Both remedies are most suitable for menopause symptoms. Salvia, or sage, is successfully used for excessive perspiration and night sweating. When the sun comes out and the temperature rises, little specks of perspiration characteristically appear on its leaves, as on the skin of a menopausal woman. Recommended use is twenty drops in some water, three times daily.

Also during question times I am often asked for reassurance that women who take HRT will not suffer from osteoporosis. This, of course, is not always true. And although HRT may help to prevent osteoporosis, a problem that affects predominantly post-menopausal women, there are other remedies that can be taken. Urticalcin is an absorbable calcium preparation from Dr Vogel and is most helpful for menopausal women. Another very useful remedy is Osteoprime, made from natural substances by Enzymatic Therapy to help prevent osteoporosis. The synthetic HRT preparation disagreed with one of my female patients, but when she started taking both these remedies she reported great improvement, which was confirmed by a scan.

I once had a middle-aged female patient who told me that she was difficult to live with as she suffered from severe mood swings which were worse in the mornings. I suggested she take Phytogen together with Female Balance, both well-tested remedies, and she became a much more pleasant person, even in the mornings.

Because of my involvement in the healthcare of

prisoners, I have met quite a number who spend time in jail for serious crimes thought to be totally out of character. Of all the prisoners I met, I'll never forget the woman who had killed her husband, not because she hated him but because she lost control, and who was full of regret and guilt. However, she could not really be held responsible for her actions at the time of the crime, because she suffered from very severe mood swings caused by hormonal imbalances. In middle age, life sometimes seems to run away with us and we can act totally out of character. This can be really frightening for many people who do not realise that something can be done to ease such symptoms. Natural remedies such as Phytogen have given lots of suffering women the help they so badly needed. Any disturbances in the hormonal balance should be rectified as soon as possible, and the means to help us achieve this are at hand.

A nationwide study looked at women who reported problems with dryness of skin, the eyes and the vagina, and insufficient replacement of the muscular layer of the fibrous tissue. This was ascribed primarily to a lack of oestrogen production. Again, a natural HRT such as Phytogen can provide help and can be used quite safely without fear of side-effects.

Sometimes depression, low blood sugar or water retention can result from low progesterone levels. This hormonal imbalance can be detrimental to a good sleeping pattern, causing fatigue, depression and inability to function. An excellent remedy in such circumstances is Hyperiforce (fifteen drops taken twice daily). Reflexology can give relief, as stimulating the feet harmonises the seven endocrine glands, while by working specifically on the pineal gland, natural Tryptophan and Melatonin will be released.

Some generally useful herbal remedies for hormonal imbalances are Dong Quai, Siberian Ginseng and Agnus castus. Diet and exercise, such as walking, cycling or swimming, are also helpful to overcome stress and disharmony in the body. Shakespeare said, 'Such harmony is in immortal souls, but while this manifesture of decay does crossly close it in, we cannot hear it.'

Our pace of life contributes to adrenal exhaustion, and reflexology, relaxation therapy and meditation can help in such situations. I have seen some lively and vibrant women change at about the age of fifty into a mere shadow of themselves. There is no need for this to happen because there are so many remedies that can take them through middle age without the lack of energy that can be caused by the menopause. At no other stage of life is hormonal balance or imbalance so telling as it is at middle age. Yet this should be a time of life to be enjoyed.

So much is written about hormones. Hormonal imbalance is always used as the reason for menstrual and pre-menstrual tension. Hormonal imbalance is the excuse for menopausal complaints in women and for the mid-life crisis in men. If we think that this is a complaint of the '70s, '80s and '90s, we are mistaken. It is simply that previously the subject was not often discussed, and even then it was only spoken about in secrecy. Recognition of the problem has only come about because of a realisation that there is no need for shame. Openness of discussion, the sharing of experiences and reading about others' problems have resulted in a very much easier situation for both men and women nowadays.

These problems do not take place in the mind, as was once thought, although the effects may manifest themselves psychologically. Such changes can happen to the most stable of characters if a mid-life crisis takes hold. This happened to a great friend of mine, and I realised that he was suffering greatly because of hormonal imbalances. I prescribed remedies and supplementary vitamins to help his immune system, and he stopped drinking. He looked at his wife with renewed interest and favourably compared her to other women to whom he had recently been attracted. Recognition of these facts saved his marriage.

Do not be too proud to seek help, because there are many good remedies available. I have recently produced a new evening primrose formula to which I have added some special ingredients which make it ideal for coping with the problems experienced during a mid-life crisis. Evening primrose oil often helps to restore hormonal balance, because in middle age essential fatty acids are often lacking in the daily diet despite being more necessary than ever.

Those of you who know me will know how much importance I attach to the endocrine system. The endocrine glands play an exceptionally important part in this period of life. Bearing in mind the three bodies of man, these glands play a major role in any hormonal imbalance. The science of endocrinology embraces the internal secretions of all the ductless glands and is something to which we ought to pay attention. The secretions from these glands discharge straight into the bloodstream and are very potent and extremely necessary to the body for its daily use. The ductless glands are the supply depot for the living organism. They regulate the nutrition we absorb from our food. Our entire physical life is regulated by these all-important glands, even down to the kind of skin or the colour of hair we have, the strength of our muscles, and so on. Many of the glands that have ducts and which form an external secretion form an internal secretion as well, i.e. liver, pancreas, the membranes of the stomach and intestines. The endocrine glands are as follows:

Pineal	Liver
Pituitary	Spleen
Carotid	Pancreas
Thyroid	Suprarenal
Parathyroids	Duodenum
Thymus	Gonads (in female)
Mammary (in female)	Prostate (in male)
Stomach	Gonads (in male)

THE PINEAL GLAND

Draw an imaginary line over the head from the top of the ears and another imaginary line from the tip of the nose to the occipital protuberance. The place where these imaginary lines cross is as close as you will get to the position of the pineal gland. There is very little known about this gland and it is often mentioned with regard to metaphysics. It is known that it secretes a fluid which assists in the growth and development of the sexual organs.

THE PITUITARY GLAND

This is localised at the nasal suture, the place where the nose meets the forehead. Just behind this junction is a saddle called the selle turica. It consists of two lobes. The *anterior* regulates the hair and fatty conditions. It is also an important factor in the growth of children. If there is an imbalance, impotence in the male and irregular periods in women can develop. It can even be the cause of excessive sugar in diabetes. The *posterior* lobe also secretes, and this acts as a tonic to the blood and is a wonderful stimulant to the intestines, promoting good digestion. Its imbalance can cause disturbances in the nervous system and digestive organs. Even low blood pressure may result, with a degree of drowsiness.

THE CAROTID GLAND

Situated directly above and a little behind the parathyroids. This gland's main importance is with regard to the sense of hearing.

THE THYROID GLAND

This is situated in front of the trachea. It influences the metabolic processes which ultimately affect the whole nervous system. It furnishes the energy to the body, without which the digestion and assimilation of food would not take place.

THE PARATHYROID GLANDS

There are four of these, situated in pairs, two on the surface of each lobe of the thyroid. These very potent secretions help the distribution of the lime salts which are essential to the body. They regulate the body weight.

Almost all other glands depend on the parathyroids for their function.

THE THYMUS GLAND

This is known as the gland of growth and is situated in the thorax, a little below the thyroid. It seems to operate until puberty Its main function is the distribution of lime to the body structure.

THE PANCREAS

This gland looks like a bunch of grapes, and is situated across the posterior wall of the abdomen. This is a gland that has an external secretion known as the pancreatic fluid. It also has an internal secretion through the islets of Langerhans. This helps to change the glucose of the blood into a form that the body tissues are able to use.

THE SPLEEN

This is situated directly below the diaphragm. Its main purpose is the regulation of the metabolic process and largely depends on the thyroid for this purpose. The spleen is related to the organs of digestion, assimilation and elimination. In an indirect way, it supplies the necessary stimulant to the stomach and intestinal tract.

THE ADRENAL GLANDS

The suprarenal and adrenal glands are small, yellowish, triangular-shaped bodies situated over each kidney. Their functions are similar and related to the autonomic nervous system, and their adrenaline secretion regulates the blood pressure.

The adrenals provide an element in the blood which

helps the process of oxidisation and thus keeps the circulation flowing at the proper pressure. If inadequate, blood pressure is often low, the nervous system is depressed and death can soon follow.

THE GONAD GLANDS

These are the reproductive organs of the body and comprise two testes in the male and two ovaries in the female. The internal secretions are poured into the blood, stimulating and revitalising all other glands and organs of the body. In co-operation with the gonads, there are the epididymis, the ductless deferens and the vesicula seminalis, as well as the ejaculatory duct and the prostate and penis. The cells (seed) in these glands emit their secretion to the body, and thus it has an external secretion.

Remember that in both mid-life crisis and menopause, reflexology, aromatherapy, osteopathy, homoeopathy and sympathy are the most helpful of therapies.

Chapter 18

REVENGE ~ FORGIVENESS

I t is good to see patients take revenge on an illness. When patients are told that there is no hope for the future, it is encouraging to see those who have a will to live refuse to accept the prognosis and start fighting their illness. This can only benefit the patient. I have seen many patients take positive revenge by fighting and overcoming their illness. On the other hand, I have also seen patients take revenge in a negative way. Having been told that they were ill, they decided that there was no point in fighting. They were the losers. In Scotland, I have often come across patients who avoided the issue by agreeing that nothing more could be done, so they take an extra dram and live life to the full – which often results in their speeding towards an untimely death.

Revenge is an emotion to be handled with care, as it can easily result in damaging attitudes or actions. I remember the battle of a very gifted singer. An HIV sufferer, he was unfortunately stricken with cancer. I watched how this man fought, and how he took revenge by positively facing his problems with great faith. In a very positive manner he changed his lifestyle. It helped that he had enormous will-power, probably due to the training and self-control that is required to be successful in his chosen profession. He positively determined to do everything possible to deal with his illness and he was widely respected and admired for the way in which he coped. Although his life was shortened because of HIV, he came to terms with his condition without giving in, and he fought a very brave battle.

Yet another patient of mine, a fellow diabetic, was told by her specialist that she should never eat a Mars bar again. Instead of listening to him she took revenge, and rather than eating one Mars bar ate three. When she came to me her kidneys had been so badly damaged by high blood pressure, largely caused by the high amount of sugar she ate, that in a very short space of time the sight in one of her eyes failed. It was useless to talk any sense to her because her revenge was directed at the specialist whose task it had been to warn her that she should never eat a Mars bar again. This is very sad, but a typical example of negative revenge. I followed in the specialist's footsteps and told her that with luck it might be possible to prevent her from losing the sight in her other eye, but only if she used her common sense and followed my advice. With the help of several natural remedies and a great deal of self-control, we managed. The damage that had already been done to cause the loss of sight in the first eye, however, could not be undone.

Not so long ago I was visited by an American musician. Years ago, when his mother was pregnant, she told me that she wanted to take revenge on her husband, who had made her pregnant against her will. She was extremely upset and irate and fully intended to terminate the pregnancy. We spoke at length and I pointed to the possible mental problems that might result, as her faith did not condone abortion. Her decision was based on revenge on her husband. Eventually she went home and, still unaware of her decision, I prayed that she would not consider solving her problems with an abortion. I never heard of her again until this young man came to see me. He had been told the story by his mother and he brought me a CD that had been recorded at a recent piano recital. He came to thank me now that he was famous and life had been so good to him. He felt that if I had not helped his mother during the difficult time of her pregnancy, he would not have been born. Her positive action prevented her from carrying out the negative revenge she had in mind.

When I see people in despair and pondering revenge, I think of the revenge planned by King Saul, when David prayed for him. At one point David tried to soften the heart of Saul by playing the harp for him, while his thoughts were centred on killing David. The music softened the mind of Saul, but his heart was so set against David that the obsession to kill him was too strong. This adversity probably gave David the strength of character he had, and in his most bitter experiences he must have remembered how God saved his life. I have often wondered why God had so much patience with David, especially when he committed an unforgivable sin. It reminds me of the great love God has for mankind, so great that whatever our sins, He will forgive and He will give us new hope and power to live our lives in better harmony. The forgiveness of God is endless, and we often do not realise how much it means to have this forgiveness and the knowledge that God has thrown our sins into this enormous ocean where they can be washed away. This is a love that is beyond human understanding.

Revenge is the opposite of forgiveness. The wife of a desperately ill patient phoned me to ask if I could give him any hope, as he did not want to live, and she was afraid that he might just slip away. His was an awkward situation because of an action that had been prejudicial to a colleague, and he feared that he would never be forgiven. I told him a story I had heard from a great friend. No matter how incredible this story may sound, it was a true story that happened some time ago. My patient listened intently. Fortunately, it helped him to regain his faith. He recovered, made a clean breast of his conscience and learned the value of forgiveness.

This is the story I told him. A railway bridge spanned a large river, and most of the day this bridge was open for shipping. It swivelled parallel with the banks to let the ships pass on both sides, because only at certain times of the day would a train come along. At those times the bridge would be turned sideways across the river, allowing the train to cross. The signalman lived in a small house at one side of the river from where he operated the controls to turn the bridge when the train approached. One evening, as the signalman was waiting for the last train, he caught sight of the train's lights in the distance. He stepped to the controls and waited for the train to be within the correct distance before he had to turn the bridge. He turned the bridge into the desired position, but to his horror he found that the locking device did not work. This was a passenger train with many people on board. At the other side of the bridge was a lever that could be used to operate the locking device manually, so he hurriedly crossed the bridge. Unless the bridge was locked securely into position, it would wobble back and forth at the end where the train approached, causing it to jump, and it might be derailed and crash into the river below. He could hear the rumble of the approaching train, took hold of the lever, leaned backwards to apply his full weight, and locked the bridge into position. He kept applying pressure to keep the mechanism locked, as so many lives depended on his strength.

Then, coming from the direction of his control cabin came a sound that made his blood run cold: 'Daddy, where are you?' His young son came across the bridge to look for him. His first impulse was to cry out to the child, but the train was already too close. The tiny legs of the boy would never be able to make it across the bridge in time. The man almost left the lever to run and snatch his son to carry him to safety, but he realised that he would not be able to get back to the lever in time. Either the passengers on the train or his young son would die. He had only a split second to reach his decision. The train sped swiftly and safely on its way and no one was even aware of the broken little body that was thrown mercilessly into the river by the onrushing train. Nor were the passengers aware of the pitiful figure of the man who stayed clinging to the lever long after the train had passed.

I asked my patient who had lost all hope for the future if he thought it was any wonder that the skies darkened and the earth trembled when God's only son died for each one of us. Nobody saw the signalman going home, walking slower than he had ever walked before, to tell his wife how he had sacrificed their son. No one can begin to comprehend the emotions that must have been in this man's heart and in the heart of his wife. One can only begin to understand a little of how God felt when he narrowed the gap between us and eternal life. As we speed through life, little time is given in thought and appreciation to Him, who sacrificed His only son in order to carry the burden of our sins. It was this story that aroused my patient who was full of remorse, and in making amends for his own misdeeds he found forgiveness.

Forgiveness is a miracle which helps us to cope with problems that could easily rob us of our health.

Chapter 19

INSOMNIA ～ MEDITATION

Counting sheep is the only way to get to sleep for some people. This is a harmless method compared to the number of pills that are taken by other people just to secure a good night's sleep. There is a huge amount of money spent in order to overcome insomnia, which is a big problem for many people. A great variety of pills are available, and it is hard to choose between them. Pillow manufacturers claim that pillows will sort out your sleeping problems, and the manufacturers of beds claim that their beds will. To some people it is extremely important which side of the bed they sleep on. No matter what, it is certain that chronic insomnia can be a very debilitating disorder with many contributing factors, including physical illness, depression and general lifestyle. Any degree of insomnia affects our health.

General advice to insomniacs is that it is wise to establish a regular bedtime and a regular time to wake up in the morning. Use the bed for sleeping, not for watching television or having midnight feasts. Avoid caffeine and alcohol for at least two hours before going to bed, do not eat a large meal late at night, and keep active during the day.

When I returned home from my first visit to Great Britain, I told my mother what a wonderful place it was because, instead of three meals a day, as we are used to in the Netherlands, I had four meals. Supper is probably one of the best meals, and is often finished with crackers and cheese. This habit does not increase the chance of a good sleep, however. Even less so does the usual cup of coffee to finish off the meal. It is much better to drink a cup of herbal tea, Melissa or peppermint tea, or any of the many herbal teas that have recently become quite popular. A walk around the garden or taking the dog for a late-evening stroll in the fresh air are good ways of preparing for the night.

Gentle exercises, as described in my book *Body Energy*, aid the release of tryptophan and melatonin, which are natural substances that encourage the endocrine system to sleep. Dormeasan, popular sleeping drops from Dr Vogel, contain a mixture of herbs that are sleep-inducing – thirty drops half an hour before going to bed will be beneficial. Valerian, which eases stress and has a mild sedative effect on the central nervous system, is also a helpful remedy. Kava-kava, a natural sedative which acts on the lymbic system of the brain, an area that regulates sleep, will also relax the central nervous system without clouding mental clarity. Kava induces feelings of peace and well-being and relaxes the muscles. Vitamins, such as B vitamins, or magnesium can also be helpful when sleeping is a problem.

It is certainly annoying when sleep will not come even though there is tiredness. The restless individual tosses from side to side, sometimes reaching for a sleeping pill – which is actually the worst action to take. If insomnia is persistent it is essential to discover and eliminate the cause. It is important what and when you eat, and if there is a history of sleeplessness, supper is the meal that ought to be forgotten.

A massage can often be very relaxing. Hydrotherapy, in the form of a brush massage with cold water, can also be useful in combination with some natural remedies. In chronic cases of sleeplessness I sometimes resort to electro acupuncture. It aims to achieve a more positive attitude and this is especially important in chronic sleep-lessness, as during the night problems tend to become insurmountable. I am very fortunate as one of the secrets of my energy is that whenever and wherever I travel, I never have any problem sleeping. Actually, sleep is my best friend, and I am fully aware that it restores my inner harmony.

A while ago a middle-aged female patient confided that after I had given her electro acupuncture treatment she had enjoyed a full night's sleep, an experience she had nearly forgotten about. She felt refreshed in the morning after a sound sleep. Life was again worth living, because she felt relaxed during the day and could cope with everything. Apart from the acupuncture treatment, I also taught her some forms of relaxation and meditation.

Meditation is a source of inner calm, and the psycho-logical effect of the power of meditation is recognised worldwide. It has proved to have a positive effect on physical health and well-being. The most significant changes are seen in slower breathing, which results in a more positive attitude to the inner self and a state of relaxation, in complete harmony with God and creation.

I have great admiration for people who have learned to meditate on the powers of God and creation and have mastered this technique. By practising these skills they have brought a calmness and an inner peace to their lives, and to the outside world they give the impression that they are at peace with themselves and creation. Meditation may appear simple, but in order to divorce oneself completely from one's surroundings it requires much practice, great will-power and strength of mind.

Many books have been written on relaxation and meditation, but it depends entirely on the individual whether or not one can learn to control the mind and meditate in calmness and in complete subjection to the will of God. In meditation there is a power of inner healing in the discovery of oneself by learning to understand the things that are out of our control. Inner harmony is essential for a balanced life.

I have already mentioned the benefits of Hara breathing exercises. One useful exercise which I will describe in more detail is a form of visualisation technique. This is ideal for the purpose of combating stress and learning to relax, and it is very useful for overcoming sleeplessness. It is also a very worthwhile exercise for people who want to come to terms with an illness and, by facing it, strengthen their determination not to succumb.

For the first part of the exercise, sit in an easy chair, with the head resting and the feet flat on the floor. Breathe calmly and listen to your breath going in and out. Now take a very deep breath and, when exhaling, tell yourself to relax. Do this three times. Then you are going to relax all the muscles of the body. Begin with the eyes and mouth. Squeeze your face tightly and suddenly let go. Feel a wave of relaxation travel down your body. Consciously tighten and then relax your neck, shoulders, arms, hands, stomach, back, upper legs, calves and feet. When you have done this, try and think of a pleasant spot where you would like to spend some time. This could be a lake, a wooded or a mountainous area. It might be your favourite holiday spot. Imagine you are there and keep the image for a few minutes. Stay there as long as you feel physically comfortable. This is a very pleasant way to induce relaxation and to combat stress.

The second part of the exercise is specifically for those coming to terms with the effects of an illness. Along with the image of a favourite place, you are now going to see your illness. You are going to see your spinal cord, this glistening white cord, the centre of all the nerves. You are going to see how bodily defences are being directed from here. You see blood vessels opening, distributing a flood of healthy blood loaded with vitamins. You see the building of cells, restoring nerves, organs and tissue. Imagine this taking place through the entire body and feel the rejuvenating effects. You may use your imagination to suit your personal circumstances, as long as you see your illness as weak and your bodily defences as strong. You are going to visualise yourself walking in beautiful countryside, without pain, feeling energetic. Breathe deeply and open your eyes.

Chapter 20

PAIN ～ COMFORT

Nobody likes to suffer pain, but pain is often the sign of an imbalance or a problem somewhere in the body, something that needs attention. Pain is an alarm bell, and if we choose to ignore the alarm, the pain will continue. There would be no pain without reason, and that applies wherever it is in the body. Looking for the cause may give some indication of how best to overcome it. See a doctor if you wish, but it is a mistake to take pain-killers, because this will only treat the symptoms and not remove the cause of the pain. Never ignore pain. Do something about it and make sure that you get some comfort or relief. There are people who grit their teeth and suffer pain, ignoring the signals, without realising that it will lead to further problems. These people need help and comfort. To receive comfort we have to understand pain, and once there is comfort, pain will often retreat. How do we derive comfort where there is pain?

Pain-control therapy has its basis in the premise that pressure on a trigger point has a healing effect, apart from its local or remote anaesthetic action. A trigger point is a sign of irritation, which is usually on the surface of the body, and can be a sign of many different diseases and pain syndromes. Firm, sustained pressure on these alarm points can check inflammation and, it is claimed, cure the disease or condition. This pressure on a trigger point, characterised by a hyper-aesthetic spot or zone of the skin, will influence the deeper organs by means of cuti-visceral reflexes.

The principle of the predominance of the cell is replaced by the idea of predominance of the autonomic nervous system. The old idea that there is no general disease, there are only diseases of the cell, must give way to the new idea that there are only general diseases. Cells and organs are only agents, as are bacteria, or the occurrence of disease and its symptoms. In this connection, the results of the research done by Dr Stoehr Jr, a physiologist, is most important, as it proves the existence of a terminal reticulum of the autonomic nervous system. It is present in all tissues and organs of the body.

Acupuncture methods, as applied by Chinese practitioners, are also based on the theoretical existence of a terminal reticulum. The nerve ends of the reticulum are interlaced to a syncytium, that is, a mass of protoplasm with numerous nuclei, forming a neural connection with the whole organism. Without the existence of a neural connection, the instantaneous peripheral reaction within an organism would be inconceivable. Examining the delicate structures of the autonomic nervous system, one may assume that the peripheral terminal of the system presents a protoplasmic texture, interpolated with nuclei. The existence of such a network is an important theoretical factor in pain control.

There are certain points in given muscles that have an area of referred pain. If one analyses these referred pains and makes gentle contact on the muscle triggers, these referred pains can be eliminated or, at least, relieved.

Remember that within every man and woman is a force which directs and controls the entire course of life. It can heal every affliction and ailment to which mankind is prone. There is continued emphasis on the importance of the blood supply to the brain, especially the emotional areas, due primarily to the excessive sympathetic stimulation of the vascular system supplying the emotional centres of the brain. In addition, this excessive stimulation causes the vessel musculature to contract, which, if prolonged, invariably produces disease. This daily bombardment of negative stimuli, the commencement of which accompanied us all from the cradle, will also persist throughout life and accompany us to the grave.

All the diseases of a given individual are spread throughout the entire organism, from the tiniest cell to the internal organs and upwards throughout the tissues. Man possesses an electrical field complete with sub-power stations and an ingenious collection of power points and fuses spread over the entire surface of the body. Visceral and body tension produce short circuits popularly known as trigger spots. Manipulation or acupuncture restore the blown fuse when a spontaneous cure usually follows. Here the sympathetic nervous system rules supreme.

From the body itself are derived the very substances essential for cure when there is illness. This simple truth, as old as mankind, has been hidden over the last couple of centuries, only to emerge again in recent years. It is acknowledged that all diseases have a common factor, and that this origin is none other than a toxaemic condition resulting from food fermentation. From the first incipient attack to the time of the cure of the patient, this original cause has a greater influence on the condition than the symptoms so frequently looked at and treated as the cause.

Comfort for pain can be given in many ways. Pain should always be investigated by a doctor or a specialist, as it indicates that there is something wrong. Never make the mistake of ignoring pain and feeling that you have to live with it.

Chapter 21

REJECTION ~ FAITH

In many of my books I have mentioned Hahnemann's principle of the three bodies. Today, more than ever before, the majority of problems arise from the third body, which is the emotional body. The emotional body can be hurt so deeply by the mental and physical bodies becoming overloaded that one may feel rejected. I feel strongly that the condition of some desperately ill patients is caused by rejection, due to misunderstanding. Certain illnesses, mental or physical, are not outwardly visible, and only too often there is a quick judgement that the patient is malingering. I am certainly against encouraging hypochondriacs or neurotics, as unfortunately there are plenty of them around. Nevertheless, I know people who have been totally rejected, by husband or wife, family or friends, because outwardly they look healthy and strong, giving the impression of robust health.

It is, of course, very easy to invent a physical condition in order to gain sympathy. I have seen this repeatedly with patients with back or neck problems. I have had patients become angry because they have been refused a doctor's certificate to sign them off work for yet another few weeks. They kept complaining about back pain, but I have treated so many people for back problems that I quickly see through such pretences. These are sad situations, made even more so because I have also had many patients who would give anything to be able to do a day's work but are too ill. Being able to work but being unwilling to do so points to rejection, and unfortunately I have seen patients who were really suffering and misunderstood, but rejected by their family.

A hospital consultant and GP had diagnosed that a young lady was suffering from ME (myalgic encephalomyelitis). ME is an ever-growing problem, and I assure you that someone suffering from a post-viral fatigue syndrome is a very ill person. The person may look well, but inside he or she will feel exhausted. ME patients often experience neck cramps, hormonal imbalances, sleeplessness during the night, sleepiness during the day, faintness and often bouts of dizziness and total exhaustion. This lady phoned me one day in tears and told me that she was about to give up because she had no strength. She felt utterly rejected and claimed that the entire village was calling her a hypochondriac behind her back. The World Health Organisation has now recognised ME, but I am disappointed because they claim that it is a problem of the mental body. I am, however, convinced that it is a problem with the immune system.

The immune system of ME patients is often so low and depleted that they are vulnerable to viruses, bacteria and parasites. When these invaders group together, their combined forces strike and expose a vulnerability in the case of low immunity. This also applies with problems such as *Candida albicans*, which is a yeast parasite. Such illnesses can take a heavy toll on a patient, and to break through and stimulate the immune system I may have to apply electro acupuncture treatment, combined with remedies such as ImunoStrength, Siberian Ginseng or enzyme products, in order to restore a balance.

With ME patients all three bodies can be under attack. ImunoStrength from Nature's Best can often provide a breakthrough, as can a number of other remedies of which the Enzymatic Therapy preparation Daily Choice Antioxidant is the best that we give to patients in the short term. I want to make it clear that it is absolutely untrue that these patients cannot be helped. It is, however, difficult to rebuild their confidence because they feel rejected and misunderstood, and mentally they may feel like outcasts in their community.

I calmly discussed these facts with this patient and assured her that life had much more to offer than rejection by unsympathetic people who did not know better. I told her that there was absolutely no need for her dejection, because I was able to help. Fortunately, she is now very much better, and is mentally, emotionally and physically overcoming her problems.

Being ill causes sufficient worry, without feeling rejection as well. Sometimes it is a question of mind, and as the mind is usually stronger than the body, patients have made themselves ill because of rejection. They feel they are living on the edge. In my book *Viruses, Allergies and the Immune System* I have written about ME and I have given plenty of evidence on how easily the immune system can be damaged and how slowly it builds up again. Eventually, however, through doing the right things, health will be restored.

People with a degenerative disease or an immune weakness often do not understand how difficult it is for a doctor, practitioner or specialist to break through to the immune system and rebuild what time has broken down. To reverse illness and disease requires time in order to rebuild and strengthen the immune system.

The immune system is a private army for battling disease and generally defending the body against countless intruders. This army is made up of various battalions of different cells with varying skills and numerous army bases and factories for the supply of all kinds of ammunition. If the soldiers are weak and unhealthy, or if the factories are short of raw materials, the army is likely to lose the battle. If the army is in good condition and well equipped, it will usually be able to fight off anything from the common cold to cholera or cancer.

The basic cause of any illness is the poor condition of the sick person's army – this is called a depressed immune system – and strengthening the immune system will often overcome the illness. A depressed immune system is recognised as the direct cause of allergies such as asthma and eczema. The condition of the immune system will, however, also affect all other illnesses, from how quickly a burn or fracture heals to how effectively a virus such as cholera is resisted. An experiment with very healthy volunteers on high-nutritional diets found that all of them, when in contact with the cholera virus, were able to fight it off quickly and easily. They did not actually contract full-blown cholera, because their immune defence armies were in excellent working order. It can be seen, therefore, that the cause of an illness is not just the existence of a condition such as a nasty bug. The cause is more often an immune system that is not working efficiently.

There are two quite different ways of dealing with an illness, the symptom-treatment approach and the cause-treatment approach. Unfortunately the symptom-treatment is the most commonly used approach, because most medical research is funded by pharmaceutical companies who can make fortunes out of treating symptoms.

If we take cancer as an example, symptom-treatment would involve attacking the cancer cells directly in order to get rid of them. This involves methods such as surgery, chemotherapy and radiation. But look at the cancer statistics for the unhappy side-effects and poor success rate of these methods. Cancers, however, are developing in our bodies most of the time. A healthy immune system will quite easily keep the cancer cells in check and destroy them. Cancer is a condition that only gets out of hand when the immune system is poor; in fact, it is actually the depressed immune system that is causing the illness. Cause-treatment, on the other hand, would build the immune system so that it could resume its work of battling with the invaders.

Of course, symptom-treatment has a place in medical

practice, but this is usually as an emergency treatment for acute symptoms. Finding the cause and clearing up the root problems tends to take longer, but cause-treatment must be implemented if the person is to become really well. For example, a malignant tumour may need to be surgically removed, but if the patient's immune system is not rebuilt the body is likely to succumb to other cancers.

Symptom-treatment often appears to give instant results. A pain-killer, for example, will cut off the pain message to the brain so that it will seem as though the problem has gone away. Of course, it has not. The body is still undergoing the shock and trauma of whatever is actually happening to cause the pain, even though the brain is not processing the information. Believing other-wise would be like being a commanding officer who, when the battle is going against him, shoots his own messengers and then celebrates a victory on the basis that no one has told him that he has lost. The cause of the pain is not being dealt with by the pain-killer. Another example is the drugs used to stop the spasms of an asthmatic lung. These can be a valuable emergency measure but do nothing to rid the body of the asthma, and further attacks can always be expected. Yet asthma can be cured.

Clearly symptom-treatment is important as an emer-gency measure, but it must not be confused with cause-treatment. Effective cause-treatment often takes time but the effects can be positive and permanent. It usually has the benefits of no side-effects, making you feel better with time, whereas symptom-treatment also has the benefits of being cheaper in the long run and of giving you the ability to take control of the problem yourself. It is sometimes fear of taking control that concerns people with little self-confidence and makes them want to leave it all to someone else. Do not be afraid. You can enjoy the challenge, and you will find that you are not on your own.

In times of war, members of our own army release a very powerful and toxic substance called histamine which is probably the most deadly of our weapons against the enemy. An antidote to this histamine, called anti-histamine, is produced by the liver to protect our own cells from being damaged by this substance. Not having the anti-histamine would be a bit like conducting chemical warfare without wearing protective clothing. If there is not enough anti-histamine to counteract all the histamine (perhaps the liver is under par, or the siege is just too great), the body does all it can to clear the toxins in other ways. Some people's bodies try to get rid of it by passing it out through the nearest mucous membrane, which becomes inflamed, as with the lungs in asthmatics or the sinuses with hay-fever sufferers. Most bodies try to deal with the problem in less obvious ways, which can have long-term and very nasty effects.

An important aspect of the warfare is, therefore, the rubbish it produces. The ability of your body to clean up the mess – dead invaders, dead defenders, chemicals of warfare waste and so on – will have a great effect on how well you conduct the next battle. A cluttered and putrefying battlefield would not be very effective.

Another source of toxins is the by-products of our bodies burning food as fuel. Our bodies need vast amounts of energy to carry out all the chemical and physical work necessary to keep us alive. The release of energy by oxidation means that the electrons, which are tiny parts orbiting each atom, leave the atom in singles and in pairs. It is like a fire with sparks flying off. The atoms which fly off are called free radicals. In a stable atom the electrons are all paired off, the negatively charged ones with the positively charged ones. However, a free radical has one spare electron which gives the atom an electrical charge so it goes off looking for something to attach to. There are those that fly off to do special jobs, mostly in the respiratory system and enzyme activity.

If the fuel is of poor quality or contaminated, various species of dangerous free radicals are produced. These can wreak havoc by attaching to stable molecules and turning them into erratic free radicals as well. A healthy body will be able to screen these free radicals and keep them under control. Most often, however, the body taking in poor fuel is also likely to have poor health, including a poor screening process. It is rather like having a screen in front of a fire to hold the sparks in check. If there are holes in the screen, or if there are just so many sparks that the screen is knocked over, the protection will be lost.

Free radicals going haywire cause havoc which is called oxy-stress. This stress influences that state of the immune system and is a major part of the ageing process. The most common form of free-radical harm is from poor-quality foods (that is, refined and processed) or rancid oils and fats. This is called lipid peroxidation and is thought to be a major factor in most age-related diseases such as arthritis, dementia and many cancers.

With such an amazingly complex immune system with all its in-built safeguards, what can possibly go wrong? Your army is most affected by three things:

1. The strength and effectiveness of the fortress walls
2. The size and strength of the foe
3. The strength of its own army

The idea of cutting down on the numbers of intruders in the body is not new. Everyday hygiene aims to do this. The problem is that we do not recognise the enemy. It is very difficult to catch anything from your cat or dog, for instance, yet you are more likely to be concerned about washing your hands after touching them than you would be about intruders from your favourite soap or chemical deodorant. These latter items, however, are likely to provide you with numerous bacteria, which the healthy body should deal with fairly easily, and chemical toxins, which your body will find much more difficult to handle.

It is estimated that on average each person in Britain consumes about 2 kg of chemical pollutants each year. Considering that only a trace of most chemicals will have profound effects, especially on the immune system, this adds up to a major attack. A body in optimum health with a regular supply of a wide range of nutrients should be able to detoxify a fair proportion of this, so if you live in a city and are subjected to petrol pollution, for example, you can minimise the damage.

I would recommend that everyone, but especially those with signs of depressed immune systems, reduce the scale of the attack by measures such as the following:

- Use only the simplest cleaning agents around the house and make sure they are environmentally friendly ones, because these will be more friendly to your body. Never use disinfectants (especially around children) and never use sprays of any sort, whether polish or perfume.
- Cut down on the amount of plastic in the environment as much as possible, because plastics constantly give off a faint gas. This includes children's toys, lunch boxes, plastic food containers and food wraps, plastic work surfaces, synthetic carpets and foam pillows.
- Be aware of and minimise your contact with items that are clearly based on chemicals that permeate your environment easily. Examples in this category would be marker pens, glues and solvents.
- Keep the home and work environment well ventilated.
- Cut out pollutants taken internally, both in food and, as much as possible, in medications. Refined sugars and caffeine, like most drugs, are very debilitating polluters. The fungicides, hormones, artificial fertilisers and other chemical pollutants in non-organically farmed fruit and vegetables make very nasty enemies. Such chemically farmed produce also tends to supply very little in the way of nutrients which would help to combat the ill effects of the pollutants. Most meat and processed foods are major sources of internal

pollution, as are food additives and processing agents. It needs to be remembered that pollutants from within the factory itself are likely to be in processed foods, especially from cleaning agents. A friend worked in a famous brewery where he nightly donned something resembling a space suit and entered enormous metal vats where he sprayed a highly toxic cleaning agent. The vats were used to make beer the next day without any attempt to rinse them.

- Most drugs and medications are very taxing on the immune system (and most other body systems). Avoid unnatural pain-killers such as aspirin and paracetamol, tranquillisers, barbiturates and so on. Find the truly helpful ways to meet your needs. Question any medications your doctor suggests and aim to understand exactly what is going on so that you can work towards cause- rather than symptom-treatment.

When your body has demands placed upon it which exceed your resources to adjust to the demands, the nervous system answers with a stress response. The chemical pathways of this stress response tend to use many parts of the body which are also crucial to the immune system, so it is not surprising that conditions of one system will affect another.

The adrenaline you tend to feel as a high is an attempt to get you ready for a 'fight or flight' situation. This hypes you up with a faster pulse, faster breathing and other effects you cannot actually see or feel. You can't feel any of the effects of the corticosteroids, but they have a tremendous impact on the immune system. One corticosteroid, called cortisol (also called hydrocortisone), will degrade tissues of the thymus gland and lymph nodes, increase T-suppressor cells while decreasing T-helper cells, and interfere with the production of the natural killer cells and interferon.

There are five aspects in building the immune system:

1. Change to a wholesome diet.
2. Exercise regularly, preferably including at least twenty minutes of aerobic exercise. Try and get at least half an hour of sunshine daily.
3. Go on an internal cleansing programme.
4. Deal with the stresses in your life.
5. Supplement your diet with a suitable range of nutrients. Each person's needs are different and you need a specialist programme drawn up by a competent naturopath or dietary consultant that will meet your particular needs. You must have advice and consult with your doctor if you are on medication. It is also necessary to consult your doctor if you have any specific disease. He may well ridicule supplementation, but he should know what may be harmful in your case.

Physical stress such as lack of sleep usually leads to emotional stress such as irritability. You can see now why emotional stress – ranging from constant negative or worrying thoughts through depression and anger to major bereavement caused by the loss of a spouse or child – will also affect the immune system and increase the chance of disease. This is why love and support from someone close makes an enormous difference to how people pull through illness. This is why sensible stress management in the workplace leads to less illness and greater achievement. This is why stress, such as that caused by bereavement, needs to be brought into the open and dealt with lovingly. It is not uncommon for one spouse to die of general poor health soon after the death of the other.

Echinacea, often described as a natural antibiotic, is an extremely effective natural preparation which stimulates the immune system in a positive way. It is a herb which the American Indians have used for a very long time for disorders relating to the immune system. Laboratory studies have confirmed that echinacea raises the white blood cell count and induces photocystosis, which means that the white blood cells increase their activities in gobbling and digesting unfriendly aliens. Many efforts have been made to identify the factors within echinacea which have immune-stimulating properties, and the controversy over which part of the plant should be isolated and made into an expensive drug continues. In the meantime, echinacea continues to be very effective. The effectiveness, however, decreases as doses get higher, until between one and three grams are taken. It is wiser to stay under one gram. Do not double up on echinacea if you are taking herbs for different reasons, such as for both immune-building and a skin disorder. Echinaforce from Dr Vogel has proved to be one of the best of the echinacea preparations.

Perhaps the most accessible – and extremely potent – immune stimulant and natural bacteriocide is the humble garlic. Its properties are so great that research papers on the topic are published with great frequency. Studies have shown that it has powerful properties for directly destroying bacteria and fungi, and that it inhibits viral multiplication. Even the HIV virus, precursor of AIDS, finds it difficult to grow in a garlic medium in tissue culture in the laboratory. It has been effectively used in the prevention of intestinal parasites, cancer of the digestive organs, and meningitis. It has now been shown, however, that garlic is able to do more than just kill micro-organisms in a safer version of an antibiotic. It also actively stimulates the immune system, especially macriphage and B-lymphocyte activity. Laboratory-isolated killer cells from garlic-eating people have been found to be much more capable of destroying tumours than the same type of cell from non-garlic consumers. There are a number of garlic supplements for those who do not eat much in their food, including the odourless version. Garlic is powerful, however, and as a supplement it should be consumed carefully, preferably with food, and at intervals.

The reason I have gone so deeply into the subject of the immune system is that in my experience people who have immunity problems often feel rejected because others do not seem to understand. It is very difficult to understand the immune system. I have great friends who have specialised in immunology, and very often they are still puzzled by it. Although many books have been published on immunity and the immune system, it is still a subject of great discussion and a diversity of opinions.

Whatever the problem, be it ME, degenerative diseases, HIV or AIDS, never feel rejected because you cannot do what others can. Have faith in the future, because some time soon help will be at hand. There are great armies working to find an answer to those problems, and brave soldiers are fighting to overcome illness and disease through faith and belief in the future.

In front of me lies a letter from a young man who always felt that faith could move mountains. This young man had a very unhappy youth with little opportunity, being rejected by his parents and growing up feeling worthless. When he was four years old he had dysentery, and at the age of seven his father left home. He told me that his diet consisted mainly of boiled eggs and fish and chips. He remembered that in his younger years he had all kinds of emotional upsets and was scared of being labelled an outcast. His nervous system was attacked, his memory failed and he had problems with his eyes. He became very depressed and later became unemployed through no fault of his own. Yet he never lost faith that he would get better. Although he had many problems, he said that through frustration he read about alternative medicines, and thanks to his own will-power he continued his efforts. After he read my book *How to Live a Healthy Life*, he knew that he should build on the three bodies of man. He had a great interest in homoeopathy and believed that natural remedies would assist him to regain health by stimulating the natural forces in his own body. He used some remedies to overcome the stress and anxiety caused by the pace and pressures of his life, and when the doctor prescribed Prozac he was happy to read in one of the national newspapers that Hyperiforce from Dr Vogel was a natural form of Prozac. He took this with the homoeopathic preparations Ignatia, Natrium mur, Aconite and Calcium carb. These remedies helped him so much that he felt greatly improved, and electro acupuncture and osteopathic manipulation concluded his treatment.

Faith can indeed move mountains, and when people lose faith, they lose everything. I remember another client of mine who had great faith in her treatment, and also in her Creator. One day when I met her on the way into the clinic, she was humming to herself. I remarked that she was rather jolly that day, and she told me that she had good reason to be happy. She explained that when she first came to me twenty-three years ago, she had been given one or two months to live, yet she is still here. She assured me that this was due to the faith she had in me, and that I had cured her. I remonstrated with her, saying that I had never cured anybody; she had cured herself because of her faith in the treatment and her undaunted faith that she would get better. It is faith that is so important. I admired the way she stuck rigidly to her treatment – and that is how I usually recognise patients who will get better. With the available techniques and the visualisation methods she practised, some from my book *Cancer and Leukaemia*, her faith was not misplaced.

This reminded me of a letter I received recently, from a lady who claimed that she had been rejected everywhere, getting the same answer all the time – that there was nothing wrong. Yet she could hardly walk. When she came to my clinic she was given manipulative treatment on her feet which actually changed her entire life, and she can now walk without pain and discomfort.

She had also been in despair about her daughter, and with her new faith in alternative treatment she managed to persuade her daughter to come and see me too. Her own successful recovery had been based on her faith, which was based on the experiences and improvement of one person only. I was worried that I might not be able to help her daughter to such improvement, but fortunately she too improved greatly.

The biggest challenge in life is to have faith in those things we cannot see, and by faith so much can be overcome. In the book of Hebrews, chapter 11:1, we read that faith is the substance of things hoped for, the evidence of things not seen. And faith does not only come from the heart. When there is faith in one's heart, there is faith in one's hands. There is so much that can be done with the hands, as I have explained in great detail in my book *Body Energy*. Energy is in the hands, and the osteopath, the reflexologist, the aromatherapist and the acupuncturist all have this tremendous power to help humanity.

Patients soon give themselves away when they enter my consulting-room by straightaway remarking on their sickness, their anxieties and their emotions, and it does a person good to unburden. To instil or encourage faith in people, I often quote the following beautiful poem:

> *Faith came singing into my room*
> *and other guests took flight,*
> *Grief and anxiety, fear and gloom,*
> *sped out into the night.*
> *I wondered that such peace could be,*
> *but Faith said gently, 'Don't you see*
> *That they can never live with me?'*

Chapter 22

DESPAIR ～ HOPE

In total despair, a young woman handed me a list. In desperation she had listed the symptoms she experienced: exhaustion, irritable bowel syndrome, stomach problems, dependency on anti-depressants, haemorrhoids, skin rashes, PMT, headaches – and at the bottom of the list was written herpes zoster virus. It was this last entry that played a major role in all the other ailments. She said that life was not worth living any more, and I was her last hope.

While she spoke I looked at her deeply in the eyes, and when she had finished her list of ailments I informed her that I had been studying her eyes to reach a diagnosis according to the iridology principle. When she told me she did not believe in iridology, I asked her what had happened to her right lung. She looked at me in disbelief and asked if I was clairvoyant. I knew that her right lung had almost collapsed, and she replied that this had been confirmed by her doctors. This quick

diagnosis, followed by her simple confirmation, initi-
ated a foundation of trust, and I promised that I would
do everything possible to help her.

What happens to people when they are in despair and
have lost all hope? It made me think of a young woman
who came to me having had a diagnosis of multiple
sclerosis confirmed. She was in a wheelchair and had
not been able to walk for some time. Over the years I
have had many MS patients under treatment and I have
seen that much can be done to control the condition,
although there is no cure. The remarkable thing was that
when this girl came to see me for the second time, she
walked into the consulting-room. It was unbelievable,
and everyone was so happy for her. On my advice she
followed a gluten-free diet, pioneered by Professor
Roger MacDougal, together with general guidelines for
MS management. She flourished on this regime. Her
own doctor was so enthusiastic that he asked her neuro-
logist for his opinion. In one breath this specialist took
away all the hope she had by telling her it was only a
remission, and the best advice he could give was to have
a stairlift installed in her house. This callous advice
destroyed all her hope. The power of hope and faith in
life was proven when she again returned to the clinic . . .
in her wheelchair.

It was a major effort to get through to her and rebuild
hope. I have always admired the view of Matthew
Henry, who said that faith, hope and charity are the
three principal graces, of which charity is the chief,
being the end to which the other two are but means.
They work together to exercise a positive attitude in the
hope that when there is mental, physical or emotional

illness, there is the hope to get better. This lady had already informed me that she prayed to God for forbearance, and I quoted her a biblical text from Exodus, chapter 15:26: 'I am the Lord and it is health I bring thee.' I told her to believe that the one who had made her healthy and who had made her walk would still take care of her. Although her belief had been shaken, I quoted an interesting passage from one of the apocryphal books, Ecclesiasticus. I lent her a copy and advised her to concentrate on verses one to fifteen of chapter thirty-eight.

Deny not a physician his due for thy need's sake; his task is of divine appointment, since from God all healing comes, and kings themselves must needs bring gifts to him. High rank his skill gives him; of great men he is the honoured guest. Medicines the most High has made of us out of earth's bounty, and shall prudence shrink from the use of them? Were not the waters of Mara made wholesome by the touch of wood? Well for us men, that the secret of virtue of such remedies has been revealed; skill the most High would impart to us, and for his marvels win renown. Thus it is that the physician cures our pain, and the apothecary makes, not only perfumes to charm the sense, but unguents remedial; so inexhaustible is God's creation, such health comes of his gift, all the world over.

Son, when thou fallest sick, do not neglect thy own needs; pray to the Lord, and thou shalt win recovery. Leave off thy sinning, thy life amend, purge thee of all guilt. With frankincense and rich oil make bloodless offering of meal; and so leave the physician to do his work. His task is of divine appointment, and thou hast need of him; let him be ever at thy side. Needs must, at times, to physicians thou shouldst have recourse; and doubt not they will make intercession with the Lord, that they may find a way to bring thee ease and remedy, by their often visiting thee. Offend thou thy maker by wrong-doing, much recourse thou shalt have to physicians.

This patient took the book home with her and my hopes were realised. At her next visit she again walked into my consulting-room, having left the wheelchair at home. With faith, prayer and meditation, despair can be overcome and transformed into that great hope that lies in the future for all of us.

The other day I received a letter from a young girl abroad, who said that nobody, including her parents, knew what had happened to her. She wrote that from the age of ten she had been emotionally, sexually and physically abused by one of her teachers, on a weekly basis, until she was seventeen years old. As is usual in these circumstances, she had been told not to tell any-body, but she needed to confide in someone. On the condition that I would tell no one and take no action, she unburdened her emotions on paper. She begged me for help. It reminded me of a similar case I had once been asked to treat, that of a teenage girl who was in the throes of a deep depression, diagnosed with all kinds of illnesses and barely able to open her eyes. She was so battered by life she had lost the will to live. Eventually I learned that at a very young age she had been raped, leaving her with physical, mental and emotional damage. The fact that she had never been able to confide in others held back her recovery. After she had spoken to me at great length, the dam burst and I detected a glimmer of hope within her. I am so proud of her because she now helps others who have lost all hope. By telling them of her own experiences she lets them know that hope must never be allowed to die, and that it lies dormant within us, even in our blackest times. A talk with a trusted friend or an encouraging remark at the right time may be all that is required for hope to spring forth again. Never give up. An understanding of what has happened helps to rebuild the house of health physically, mentally and emotionally.

On my travels I met a lady who knew the depth and the measure of despair. Her life story was something she asked me never to speak about. I listened to her, and in time she slowly fought her way back from the brink of despair. That she turned the corner is clear from the poem she sent me, which I use with her permission.

THE MEASURE

Upon what scale can greatness be measured?
Do we look into the haughty face of the wealthy man
Whose life is entwined in conspicuous consumption
Who although his pockets be full
His heart is empty and barren
And his soul an ice cavern lined all in cold blue
diamonds
So when he screams into its empty void
He hears only the echoes of his own folly calling back

Or is greatness measured by that lofty position
Reserved only for the powerful
Can eminence be detected in aristocratic arrogance
As it swings its purple cape
Digging its heavy footsteps into the backs
Of those whom it would make its stairwell
On a useless venture
To the peaks of despair
And what of the view from on high
Are the clouds the focus of his gaze
Or are the jagged cliffs below his fate
As they lay in wait with angry sharp jaws
For that one fatal slip of his haughty foot
Or is greatness reflected in the eyes of the man
Who strives forward with all the integrity of his spirit
To attain perfection so that he can share
His excellence with his fellow wanderers upon this earth
So that he can swing his garden gate wide to them
And never weary of the lost and wandering
By this man can greatness be truly measured
And his light shines luminously
Through this dark and stormy world.

If everything seems lost and all hope is gone, pick up the threads and see how despair can be moved aside by hope. Never give up hope of getting better. I want to emphasise this by quoting part of a letter I received from the girl with herpes zoster virus whom I mentioned at the beginning of this chapter.

> I really want to thank you from the bottom of my heart for the miracle of making me better. I had this

dreadful virus for eight years and believed that I would have to live with it forever. I am so happy and feel released from the shame and anxiety that came with it. Not an hour passed in the 'old days' without me thinking about it. Now I don't give it a thought.

Despite seeing much misery and despair in my work, hope lives eternally, fuelled by letters from patients expressing their gratitude and appreciation. I quote from another patient's letter of hope.

I felt I would like to write to you a note of our expression of sincere gratitude for your caring on behalf of my husband and self. You give such hope and upliftment to your patients and give faith and hope to so many who feel despairing. No doubt you receive the praise you deserve for your dedication in your life's work. You have a wonderful understanding of Mother Nature and creation and are so greatly 'in tune' with nature and beauty, enabling you to be attuned to natural remedies for wellbeing.

This lady signed her letter 'With sincerity of heart', and this is what counts when the heart is in it, the whole body is in it. We either want to share our lives with others or give ourselves with heart and soul to what we are doing. I say again that often, when all seems lost, there is still hope.

I think of a great sportsman, to whom sport was everything, a way of life. He had been earmarked for a great future in his chosen sport, but because of injuries his career looked to be short-lived. All his dreams were centred on his sport, with the result that he lost all hope for the future. Through successful treatment he grew physically strong again, his hope re-emerged and he became one of the greatest sportsmen in his chosen sport. It was the hope and the faith he had after he had got better physically that gave him back the belief in himself and his abilities.

I always remember one of my professors telling me that the Bible, the most widely read book on earth, starts in a garden and ends in a city. It is a building process, and that is what life is about. Build on oneself and build on one's health, never despair of getting better, and never give up hope. Sometimes it is necessary to dig deep, and I remember an elderly man who made a great impression on me when I was still quite young. This man told me that in his first job after he had chosen to become a gardener, he understandably knew very little about the work that was entrusted to him. When his boss gave him some seeds to plant, he was so happy when the seedlings sprouted. He nursed them in the sunshine and delighted in the way they flourished. When he thought they were ready for planting out, his boss took the trays and put them in a dark cellar with only a little water. Not until he thought that they were nearly dead was he told to plant them in the garden. They became wonderfully strong plants, and the gardener had learned the lesson that because they had experienced hardship they had gone on to achieve great strength.

So it is in life. Physically, mentally and emotionally,

we should be hardened to all conditions. A five-year-old girl walked into my consulting-room and gave me a hug. She is a sweet little thing, but her life will not be long because she has an inoperable tumour. Yet, with her enormous zest for life, she fights, with the full support and encouragement of her parents.

While I am writing this book I look at an invitation from an American patient to attend a party. She was told nearly seven years ago at a leading London hospital that she might have only one month to live. An inoperable tumour had been diagnosed. She had great faith, great hope and a strong desire to make the best of it. With delight, I read her letter inviting all those who helped her to a celebration party, since the hospital has now confirmed that she is completely well. She used all means to fight the tumour, and was helped by a strong immune system and her great faith in Him who gave her life, and has given it back again. Now she wanted to share with others who may be in need of help.

In this world full of destruction, pain and misery, there is still great hope for the future. While closing this book I look from my attic room over the sea, towards the island of Arran. The sun is sinking, giving a beautiful warm glow over the sea, and everything looks peaceful. The earthly city of Jerusalem was the city of God's tears. The new and heavenly Jerusalem will be the city of His throne, as mentioned in the last chapter of the Bible. The one who wept over the earthly Jerusalem (Luke 19:44) will be the same one who will wipe away all tears from our eyes in that heavenly Jerusalem, and in that city no one will ever weep again.

What a comfort it is to know that our pain- and fear-ridden world will one day be free of all these destructive forces, but while we are in this life let us make the very best of it, and let us use the gifts God has given us to help each other through this life, to make it as happy and as healthy as possible. From a colleague of mine, Joyce Poley, I received a song, the words of which I use in conclusion of this book.

HANDS OF THE HEART

Deep in our soul lie feelings and plans
Waiting to dance into life through our hands
The poet writes sonnets
The artist paints dreams
And all of our world becomes more than it seems.

And we touch one another in our own special way
In a letter of love or a sculpture of clay
In the squeeze of a hand or a gentle caress
And the more we reach out, the more we are blessed.

Each of us shares who we are through our hands
In playing concertos or tilling the land
In a doll stitched with care or a great work of art
Our hands are the tools that speak for the heart.

APPENDICES

BIBLIOGRAPHY

Chappell, Peter, *Emotional Healing and Homoeopathy*, Element Publishing, Shaftesbury, Dorset, Rockport, USA

Clement, Briand and Anna Maria, *Relationships*, AM Press, West Palm Beach, Florida, USA

Ford, David F., *The Shape of Living*, Fount Harpers, Collins, Glasgow, UK

Humphreys, Tony, *The Power of Negative Thinking*, Gill and MacMilland, London, UK

Kubler-Ross, Elizabeth, *To Live Until We Say Goodbye*, Prentice Hall Inc, Englewood, Cliffs, USA

Lewis, C.S., *The Four Loves*, Collins, Glasgow, UK

Meares (MD), Ainsley, *Relief Without Drugs*, Souvenir Press, UK

Russel, Lao, *God Will Work With You, But Not For You*, University of Science, Swannanova, Virginia, USA

Vegotsky, Ken, *Make Love With Life*, Ages Publications, Toronto, Canada

Vogel, Alfred, *The Nature Doctor*, A Vogel Verlag, Teufen, Switzerland

Westlake, Aubrey, *The Pattern of Health*, Vincent Stuart, London, UK

Woodward, Christopher, *A Doctor Heals By Faith*, Max Parish, London, UK

USEFUL ADDRESSES

Auchenkyle
Southwoods Road, Troon, Ayrshire KA10 7EL

Bach Flower Remedies
Unit 6, Suffolk Way, Abingdon, Oxon OX14 5JX

Bioforce Canada Ltd
11 German Street, Newmarket, Ontario L3Y 7V1

Bioforce UK Ltd
2 Brewster Place, Irvine, Ayrshire KA11 5DD

Bioforce USA Ltd
Kinderhook, New York, USA

Britannia Health Products Ltd
Forum House, Brighton Road, Redhill, Surrey RH1 6YS

British Acupuncture Association
34 Alderney Street, London SW1V 4EU

Enzymatic Therapy (UK)
Hadley Wood Healthcare, 28 Crescent West, Hadley
 Wood, Barnet, Herts EN4 0EJ

Enzymatic Therapy (USA)
PO Box 22310, Green Bay, W1 54305, USA

General Council and Register of Osteopaths
56 London Street, Reading, Berks RG1 4SQ

Hadley Wood Healthcare
28 Crescent Way, Hadley Wood, Barnet, Herts EN4 0EJ

Nature's Best
Dept HT01, 1 Lamberts Road, Tunbridge Wells, Kent
 TH2 3EQ

A. Nelson & Co. Ltd
5 Endeavour Way, Wimbledon, London SW19 9UH

INDEX